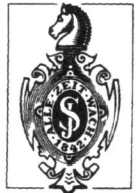

W. Kleine H.-G. Meerpohl
A. Pfleiderer Ch. Z. Profous (Hrsg.)

Therapie des Endometriumkarzinoms

Mit 15 Abbildungen
und 39 Tabellen

AGO
Arbeitsgemeinschaft für
Gynäkologische Onkologie

Springer-Verlag
Berlin Heidelberg New York
London Paris Tokyo
Hong Kong Barcelona
Budapest

Priv.-Doz. Dr. med. Werner Kleine
Priv.-Doz. Dr. med. Hans-Gerd Meerpohl
Prof. Dr. med. Albrecht Pfleiderer

Universitäts-Frauenklinik
Hugstetter Straße 55
W-7800 Freiburg

Dr. Christian Z. Profous

Farmitalia Carlo Erba GmbH
Merzhauser Straße 112
W-7800 Freiburg

ISBN-13:978-3-540-54571-2   e-ISBN-13:978-3-642-76950-4
DOI: 10.1007/978-3-642-76950-4

Die Deutsche Bibliothek - CIP-Einheitsaufnahme
Therapie des Endometriumkarzinoms: mit 39 Tabellen / AGO - Arbeitsgemeinschaft für
Gynäkologische Onkologie. W. Kleine ... (Hrsg.). - Berlin; Heidelberg; New York; London;
Paris; Tokyo; Hong Kong; Barcelona; Budapest: Springer 1991
ISBN-13:978-3-540-54571-2
NE: Kleine, Werner [Hrsg.]; Arbeitsgemeinschaft für Gynäkologische Onkologie

Dieses Werk ist urheberrechtlich geschützt. Die dadurch begründeten Rechte, insbesondere
die der Übersetzung, des Nachdrucks, des Vortrags, der Entnahme von Abbildungen und
Tabellen, der Funksendung, der Mikroverfilmung oder der Vervielfältigung auf anderen
Wegen und der Speicherung in Datenverarbeitungsanlagen, bleiben, auch bei nur auszugs-
weiser Verwertung, vorbehalten. Eine Vervielfältigung dieses Werkes oder von Teilen dieses
Werkes ist auch im Einzelfall nur in den Grenzen der gesetzlichen Bestimmungen des Urheberrechtsgesetzes der Bundesrepublik Deutschland vom 9. September 1965 in der jeweils
geltenden Fassung zulässig. Sie ist grundsätzlich vergütungspflichtig. Zuwiderhandlungen
unterliegen den Strafbestimmungen des Urheberrechtsgesetzes.

© Springer-Verlag Berlin Heidelberg 1991

Die Wiedergabe von Gebrauchsnamen, Handelsnamen, Warenbezeichnungen usw. in
diesem Werk berechtigt auch ohne besondere Kennzeichnung nicht zu der Annahme, daß
solche Namen im Sinne der Warenzeichen- und Markenschutz-Gesetzgebung als frei zu
betrachten wären und daher von jedermann benutzt werden dürfen.

Produkthaftung: Für Angaben über Dosierungsanweisungen und Applikationsformen
kann vom Verlag keine Gewähr übernommen werden. Derartige Angaben müssen vom
jeweiligen Anwender im Einzelfall anhand anderer Literaturstellen auf ihre Richtigkeit
überprüft werden.

Satz und Layout: Reiner Göhrick, Manuskript- & Textverarbeitung, 7630 Lahr

Vorwort

Das Endometriumkarzinom ist heute das häufigste Genitalkarzinom der Frau. Eine Fülle von neuen Erkenntnissen über die Ausbreitung und die Prognosefaktoren des Endometriumkarzinoms sowie mehrere große Studien haben zu einer neuen Sicht der Therapie dieses Karzinoms geführt. Die routinemäßige Lymphonodektomie steht zur Diskussion und damit die Ausdehnung der Operation bei prognostisch ungünstigen Fällen und die Einschränkung der Radikalität bei prognostisch günstigen. Früher routinemäßig durchgeführte Maßnahmen wie die Strahlen- und die Gestagentherapie werden in Frage gestellt. Dieser Wandel der Vorstellungen in der Behandlung des Endometriumkarzinoms ließ es notwendig erscheinen, in einem kleinen Kreis international bekannter Experten, den aktuellen Stand der Therapie des Endometriumkarzinoms neu zu diskutieren. Dazu hatte die Arbeitsgemeinschaft für gynäkologische Onkologie der Deutschen Krebsgesellschaft und der Deutschen Gesellschaft für Geburtshilfe und Gynäkologie zu einem Symposium im August 1990 nach Freiburg eingeladen.

Die wichtigsten Referate dieses Symposiums wurden ausgearbeitet und können jetzt mit Unterstützung der Firma Farmitalia Carlo Erba GmbH, Freiburg publiziert werden. Das Symposium verlief in englischer Sprache. Um die Akzeptanz im deutschsprachigen Raum zu erhöhen, waren die deutschen Autoren gehalten, ihren Beitrag in Deutsch abzufassen. Während die Beiträge aus dem englischen Sprachraum im Original übernommen wurden.

Der Band über die »Therapie des Endometriumkarzinoms« ergibt so einen aktuellen Überblick über die Wandlungen und neuen Entwicklungen bei der Therapie des Endometriumkarzinoms. Er wendet sich an alle Gynäkologen, an alle gynäkologischen Onkologen und alle Onkologen, die an der Therapie des Endometriumkarzinoms interessiert sind.

Freiburg im Mai 1991

Prof. Dr. A. Pfleiderer   Priv. Doz. Dr. W. Kleine

Inhaltsverzeichnis

Vorwort V

I. Einführung

Möglichkeiten und Probleme der Diagnostik
und Therapie des Endometriumkarzinoms
A. Pfleiderer 3

II. Prognosefaktoren

Histopathology of Endometrial Cancer
H. Fox 25

Östrogen- und Progesteronrezeptoren
beim Endometriumkarzinom
W. Kleine 31

Estrogen and Progestin Receptors
in Relation to Conventional Prognosis
Indicators in Endometrial Carcinomas
A. Kauppila 43

Flow Cytometry in Invasive Endometrial
Carcinoma
C. Tropé, J. Kaern, B. Lindahl, and I. Vergote 53

Oncogenes in Endometrial Cancer:
A Review of Information
E.I. Kohorn, B.M. Kacinski 58

EGF Receptor (EGF-R)
Analysis in Endometrial Carcinomas
T. Bauknecht 65

On Hereditary Factors in Endometrial Carcinoma
S. Kullander 76

III. Operatives Vorgehen

Surgery for Endometrial Carcinoma
N.F. Hacker 83

Treatment of Clinical Early Endometrial
Carcinoma; Indications for Lymphonodectomy
J. Aalders 91

IV. Radiotherapie

Postoperative Vaginal Irradiation
by High-Dose-Rate Cobalt Afterloading
in Stage I Endometrial Cancer: Experience
from the Norwegian Radium Hospital
I. Vergote, K. Kjorstad, V. Abeler, and S. Vossli 103

V. Hormontherapie

Adjuvante Hormontherapie beim Endometriumkarzinom
M. Kaufmann 111

Palliative Hormonal Treatment
in Endometrial Carcinoma
K.-D. Schulz, J. Hofmann, R. Hackenberg, G. Emons,
P. Schmidt-Rhode, and G. Sturm 119

VI. Chemotherapie

Systemic Chemotherapy for Advanced
or Recurrent Endometrial Cancer
H.-G. Meerpohl 133

Autorenverzeichnis

Aalders J.G., Prof.
Department of Obstetrics and University Hospital
Oostersingel 59 Groningen
Postbus 30.001
NL - 9700 RB Groningen, Netherlands

Bauknecht T., PD Dr. med.
OA der Universitäts-Frauenklinik
Hugstetter Straße 55
D-7800 Freiburg, Germany

Fox H., Prof., Dir.
University of Manchaster
Department of Pathological Sciences
Oxford Road
Manchaster M 13 9 PT, United Kingdom

Hacker N.F., Prof.
Dep. of Gynecologic Oncology
Royal Hospital for Women
University of New South Wales
Sydney, Australia

Kaufmann M., Prof. Dr. med.
Ltd. OA der Universitäts-Frauenklinik
Voßstr. 9
D-6900 Heidelberg, Germany

Kaupilla A., Prof.
Dep of Obstetrics and Gynecology
University of Oulu,
SF-90220 Oulu, Finland

Kleine W., PD Dr. med.
OA der Universitäts-Frauenklinik
Hugstetter Str. 55
D-7800 Freiburg, Germany

Kohorn E.I., Prof. M. D.
Yale University, Dep of Obstet. Gynecol.
Medical School
339 F. P.O. Box 3333
New Haven – CT 06510, USA

Kulander Stig, Prof. M. D.
Dep of Obstetrics and Gynecology
University of Lund
S-21401 Malmö, Sweden

Meerpohl H.-G., PD Dr. med.
OA der Universitäts-Frauenklinik
Hugstetter Str. 55
D-7800 Freiburg, Germany

Pfleiderer A., Prof. Dr. med.
Geschäftsführender Direktor der
Universitäts-Frauenklinik
Hugstetter Str. 55
D-7800 Freiburg, Germany

Schulz K.-D., Prof. Dr. med.
Geschäftsführender Direktor der
Universitäts-Frauenklinik
Pilgrimstein 3
D-3550 Marburg, Germany

Tropé C., Prof.
The Norwegian Radium Hospital
Dep of Gynecologic Oncology
Montebello
N-3010 Oslo 3, Norway

Vergote I., M. D.
 The Norwegian Radium Hospital
 Dep of Gynecologic Oncology and Pathology
 Montebello
 N-0310 Oslo 3, Norway

I. Einführung

Möglichkeiten und Probleme der Diagnostik und Therapie des Endometriumkarzinoms*

Albrecht Pfleiderer

Hier wird versucht, die wichtigsten Publikationen und Erkenntnisse aus den Jahren 1989 und 1990 zum Thema Endometriumkarzinom zu referieren, um so einen aktuellen Überblick über die Diagnostik und die Therapie dieses Karzinoms im August 1990 zu fixieren.

A. Zwei Formen des Endometriumkarzinoms

Das Endometriumkarzinom gilt unter den gynäkologischen Karzinomen als relativ harmlos, da 74% im Stadium I diagnostiziert werden und 72% von diesen 5 Jahre überleben. Die Heilungsrate liegt sogar bei 90%, wenn man nur 30 bis 69 Jahre alte Frauen berücksichtigt, die operiert wurden [2]. Dies betrifft jedoch nur zwei Drittel aller Patientinnen mit einem Endometriumkarzinom. Über 30% der Patientinnen werden an diesem Karzinom sterben. Vieles spricht dafür, daß man zwei pathogenetisch verschiedene Typen unterscheiden muß [6,30]. Der eine Typ, Typ A, ist charakterisiert durch das sog. »Korpuskarzinomsyndrom«: Fettsucht, Hyperlipidämie, Diabetes und Infertilität. Diesem Karzinom gehen hyperplastische Prozesse im Endometrium und nicht selten eine langdauernde Östrogenzufuhr voraus. Das Tumorgewebe ist durch einen hohen Progesteron- und Östrogenrezeptorgehalt charakterisiert. Die Prognose dieser Karzinome ist sehr gut. Der andere Typ, Typ B, läßt alle diese Kennzeichen vermissen: Progesteronrezeptoren sind nur schwach oder nicht vorhanden, das Karzinom ist entdifferenziert, im Myometrium tief invasiv, neigt zu Lymphknotenmetastasen und hat eine sehr ungünstige Prognose.

---

* Herrn Prof. Wenz zum 65. Geburtstag in kollegialer Freundschaft, verbunden mit dem Wunsch einer weiterhin vertrauensvollen Zusammenarbeit

Die Methoden der Früherkennung haben sich bisher nur auf den Typ A konzentriert. Es kann deshalb nicht verwundern, daß sich mit der Beherrschung der postoperativen Mortalität und dem Wegfall des Lokalrezidivs durch die Operation, an der eigentlichen Heilungsrate dieses Karzinoms weltweit seit 1962 fast nichts mehr geändert hat [2]. Dieses Dilemma resultiert wahrscheinlich daraus, daß sich an der Prognose der malignen Formen nichts geändert hat. Um dieses Problem zu lösen, sind für die Fälle des Typ B neue Strategien der Früherkennung und Behandlung nötig.

B. Früherkennung durch Vaginosonographie

Mit der Vaginosonographie ist es möglich, Strukturen im kleinen Becken sehr viel präziser zu erkennen als mit der Abdominalsonographie. Das gilt besonders für das Uteruscavum und die Adnexgegend. Osmers u.a.[28] berichten über die Vaginosonographie bei 103 postmenopausalen Patientinnen mit atypischen Blutungen und bei 283 Frauen ohne diese. Alle diese Patientinnen wiesen in der Adnexgegend keine tastbaren Tumoren auf und hatten die typische hormonale, postmenopausale Situation mit niedrigen Östrogenen und hohem FSH. Die Autoren maßen die Dicke des Endometriums und verglichen das Ergebnis mit der histologischen Untersuchung. Bei der Gruppe mit postmenopausaler Blutung war das Endometrium in 45% der Fälle nur 1-3 mm dick und enthielt weder eine atypische adenomatöse Hyperplasie noch ein Karzinom. In 55% (57 Fälle) war das Endometrium dicker als 4 mm. Es enthielt in 23% ein Endometriumkarzinom, in 9% eine atypische adenomatöse Hyperplasie und in weiteren 9% andere maligne Tumoren. Von den 283 asymptomatischen Patientinnen wurden alle die Frauen kürettiert, bei denen das Endometrium mehr als 4 mm dick war. Bei diesen 45 Frauen fand sich in 10 Fällen ein Endometriumkarzinom, in 2 Fällen eine atypische adenomatöse Hyperplasie und in 3 Fällen ein anderer maligner Tumor. Insgesamt fand sich bei 12,6% aller Frauen mit postmenopausaler Blutung und bei 3,5% aller symptomfreien postmenopausalen Frauen ein Endometriumkarzinom. Diese Frequenz ist höher als die, die bei der US-National-Endometrium-Study (1981) entdeckt wurde [23]. Bemerkenswert ist dabei die relativ geringe Rate einer atypischen adenomatösen Hyperplasie, von der sich nur 7 Fälle im Vergleich zu 23 Endometriumkarzinomen fanden. Die niedrige Rate an Präkanzerosen gibt einen Hinweis darauf, daß mit der Methode der Vaginosonographie, wie zu erwarten, auch Karzinome entdeckt werden, denen die typischen Risikofaktoren fehlen.

C. Prognosefaktoren des Endometriumkarzinoms

1. Karzinom oder atypische adenomatöse Hyperplasie?

Ob ein atypisches Endometrium nur in sich atypisch ist oder auch invasiv wächst und damit ein Karzinom ist, ist am Abrasionsmaterial oft kaum zu entscheiden. Fehlinterpretationen sind häufig. Lee and Scully [24] berichten über 10 Fälle von Patientinnen unter 21 Jahren mit der Diagnose »schwere atypische endometriale Hyperplasie oder Karzinom«, die Scully in 17 Jahren gesammelt hatte. Bei 9 dieser 10 Fälle war die ursprüngliche Diagnose Karzinom gewesen. Lee und Scully [24] konnten diese Diagnose aber nur in 4 Fällen bestätigen. Bei jungen Patientinnen ist die Tendenz groß, schwere Grade der Hyperplasie überzubewerten. Wenn die proliferierenden Drüsen nicht zusammenfließen, wenn keine Stromareaktion besteht und keine Kernatypien vorhanden sind, handelt es sich auch um kein Karzinom. Keine dieser 10 Patientinnen und keine andere Patientin mit einem hochdifferenzierten Endometriumkarzinom unter 21 Jahren ist nach Berichten in der Literatur an ihrem Karzinom verstorben oder entwickelte Metastasen. In der überwiegenden Mehrzahl aller Fälle ist es deshalb gerechtfertigt, nicht nur auf alle adjuvanten Maßnahmen zu verzichten, sondern insbesondere den Uterus zu erhalten. Eine mehrjährige Gestagenbehandlung, die allerdings über 2–3 Jahre dauern sollte, führt nach allen bisherigen Informationen zur Heilung und erlaubt nachfolgende Schwangerschaften.

2. Ungünstige histologische Subtypen

Bekanntlich unterscheiden sich seröse, hellzellige und adenosquamöse Endometriumkarzinome grundsätzlich von den typischen sogenannten endometrioiden Adenokarzinomen des Endometriums. Wilson u.a. [43] berichten über 388 Patientinnen, die wegen eines Endometriumkarzinoms von 1979–1983 in der Mayo-Klinik in Rochester USA behandelt worden waren. Darunter waren 20 (5%) adenosquamöse, 14 (4%) serös-papilläre, 11 (3%) hellzellige und 7 (2%) undifferenzierte Karzinomfälle. Im Gegensatz zur 5-Jahresüberlebensrate der Patientinnen mit endometrioiden Karzinomen (92%) lag die 5-Jahresüberlebensrate aller Subtypen zusammen bei nur 33%. Die Arbeit bestätigt damit frühere Analysen. Interessant ist aber, daß nur 17% dieser Patientinnen über eine exogene Östrogenbehandlung berichteten im Vergleich zu 29% bei Patientinnen mit endometrioidem Adenokarzinom. Bei chirurgischem Staging (neue Stadieneinteilung) waren nur 37% der Fälle mit ungünstigem Subtyp auf das Corpus uteri (Stadium I) beschränkt, verglichen mit 87% beim endometrioiden Typ. 62% entfielen auf die neuen FIGO-Stadien III und IV, verglichen mit 7% beim endometrioiden Typ. Die ungünstigen Typen wurden in 73% als Broders-Grad III und IV, (verglichen mit 11% beim endometrioiden Typ) eingeteilt und wiesen in 44% (verglichen mit 3%) eine Tumorpenetration durch die Uterusserosa auf. 55% hatten Metastasen außerhalb der Bauchhöhle und des kleinen Beckens. Trotz großzügiger Indikationsstellung zu postoperativer Strahlentherapie in 56%, Gestagenbehandlung in 17% und Chemotherapie in 8%, überlebten von den adjuvant behandelten Patientinnen nur 10% 5 Jahre. Diese Untersuchung, die insgesamt bekannte Daten bestätigt, ist insofern bemerkenswert, als die Inzidenz der ungünstigen Subtypen relativ niedrig ist und deren Überlebensraten schlechter als in allen anderen entspechenden Serien. Dies gibt einen Hinweis auf die exzellente Selektion und das hohe maligne Potential dieser Tumoren.

3. Rezeptorstatus

Beim Endometriumkarzinom scheint, verglichen mit dem Mammakarzinom, was den Rezeptorstatus anbetrifft, eine andere Situation vorzuherrschen. Die Expression des Epidermal-Growth-Factor-Receptor (EGF-R) ist beim Mammakarzinom mit schlechter Prognose und invers zur Expression des Östrogenrezeptors korreliert [3,36]. In normal proliferierendem und sekretorischem Endometrium ist der EGF-R stärker exprimiert als im endometrioiden Adenokarzinom. Eine Beziehung zwischen EGF-R und anderen Prognosefaktoren oder zum Östrogenrezeptor-Status war nicht festzustellen [3,5].

Die vermutete Korrelation zwischen Östrogen- und Progesteronrezeptorstatus auf der einen und der Prognose des Endometriumkarzinoms auf der anderen Seite [12,20,21,30] kann heute als gesichert gelten. Eine der größten Untersuchungen, die sich (zum ersten Mal) auf die echte 5-Jahresüberlebensrate bezieht, wurde jetzt von Kleine u.a.[22] publiziert.

Eine multivariate Analyse an 283 Endometriumkarzinomen einschließlich 38 Rezidivfällen und 26 Sarkomfällen des Endometriums beweist den Progesteronrezeptor mit einem cut off-point von 50 fmol als unabhängigen Prognosefaktor. In seiner Validität ist er nach dem klinischen Stadium der stärkste Prognosefaktor. Im Vergleich dazu haben der Östrogenrezeptor (cut off-point 50 fmol) und der Differenzierungsgrad allein keine signifikante prognostische Bedeutung. In einer retrospektiven Analyse gestagen-behandelter Fälle (16 adjuvant und 17 palliativ) konnten Kleine u.a. [22] zeigen, daß, was das Überleben betrifft, ein relevanter Unterschied zwischen Progesteron-Rezeptor-positivem und Rezeptor-negativem Endometriumkarzinom, nicht aber zwischen behandelten und unbehandelten Patientinnen besteht. Die Analyse ergibt weiterhin, daß in Rezidivtumoren und in Fernmetastasen Progesteronrezeptoren nur in höchstens einem Drittel aller Fälle vorkommen. Zu ähnlichen Zahlen kommen Borazjani u.a. [8].

4. Zellkinetische Parameter

Die prognostische Bedeutung des DNA-Index, bestimmt durch Flow-Zytophotometrie an frischem Material, ist etabliert [16,26]. Der DNA-Gehalt hat sich als ein besserer Parameter erwiesen als alle anderen bekannten Prognosefaktoren. Nach Lindahl u.a. [26] kann man die Endometriumkarzinome in 3 Gruppen einteilen:

1. Diploide Karzinome mit einer Rezidivrate von 6%.

2. Aneuploide Karzinome mit hohem Östrogenrezeptor und ohne tiefe myometrane Invasion mit einer Rezidivrate von 18%.

3. Aneuploide Karzinome mit niedrigem Östrogenrezeptor und tiefer myometraner Invasion mit einer Rezidivrate von 44%.

Die Methode ist an Paraffin eingebettetem Material ebenfalls möglich. Britton u.a.[9] analysierten Archivpräparate von 203 Patientinnen mit Endometriumkarzinom im chirurgischen Stadium I (neue FIGO-Klassifikation), die in der Mayo-Klinik 1979-1983 behandelt worden waren. Sie fanden bei 84% der Fälle ein diploides DNA-Muster, bei 3% ein tetraploides und bei 12% ein aneuploides. Die diploiden Fälle rezidivierten in 6%, die nicht-diploiden in 31%. Unabhängig von der Behandlung oder anderen pathologischen Kriterien wie Differenzierungsgrad und Subtyp betrug das progressionsfreie 5-Jahresintervall (Kaplan-Meier) für die diploiden Karzinome 92%, für die nicht-diploiden 63%. Von 7 Fällen mit Tumorzellen in der Peritoneallavage (beim Stadium I, chirurgisch) waren 2 nicht-diploid, die beide rezidivierten, und 5 diploid, die alle nicht rezidivierten. Die DNA-Ploidie läßt sich am Abrasionsmaterial messen. Damit läßt sich schon präoperativ eine Aussage über die Prognose des Tumors machen. Rosenberg u.a. [35] bestätigten diese Resultate und zeigten darüberhinaus, daß Karzinome mit einer S-Phase-Fraktion unter 5% in 5 Jahren eine kumulative Mortalität von 7%, solche mit über 10% S-Phasen-Anteil dagegen eine Mortalität von 49% aufweisen.

D. Das Problem der Stadieneinteilung

1. Die neue FIGO-Klassifikation 1988

Die Stadieneinteilung des Endometriumkarzinoms erfolgte bekanntlich bisher ausschließlich klinisch. Die Resultate sind bekannt und fanden weithin Verbreitung [2]. Die Stadieneinteilung ließ sich für Operierte und Nichtoperierte gleichermaßen anwenden. Das hatte insofern Bedeutung, als der Prozentsatz der primären Hysterektomie beim Endometriumkarzinom früher bei etwa 50% lag. Heute werden dagegen über 90% aller Fälle mit einem Endometriumkarzinom im klinischen Stadium I hysterektomiert (Tabelle 1). Im Oktober 1988 änderte das FIGO-Komitee für gynäkologische Onkologie in Rio de Janeiro die Stadieneinteilung grundlegend. Ab jetzt soll die Einteilung pathologisch-anatomischen Gesichtspunkten folgen und damit ausschließlich auf Grund des postoperativen Status und der histologischen Untersuchung vorgenommen werden (Tabelle 2).

Um die beiden Einteilungen vergleichen zu können, analysierten wir retrospektiv das prä- und das postoperative Staging für alle Fälle, die bei uns 1979-1988 behandelt wurden (Tabelle 3). Vergleicht man die beiden Klassifikationen an den gleichen Fällen (Tabelle 4), so ergeben sich in allen Stadien andere 5-Jahresüberlebensraten. Die Ergebnisse sind in den Stadien I, III und IV besser, im Stadium II schlechter. Dabei ist erstmals der Unterschied zwischen den Stadien I und II signifikant. Um exakte Daten zu bekommen und um günstige und ungünstige Fälle besser zu unterscheiden, ist diese neue Form des Stagings unseres Erachtens unverzichtbar.

In der abrupten Änderung des Stagings liegt jedoch eine Fülle ungelöster Probleme. Die wichtigsten seien hier kurz aufgeführt:

Erstens: Inoperable Fälle können nicht entsprechend eingeteilt werden.
Zweitens: Die präoperative Bestrahlung, die in vielen Institutionen mit guten Resultaten vorgenommen wurde [14], ist nicht mehr möglich (vergleichbar).
Drittens: Die Berücksichtigung von Lymphknotenmetastasen (Stadium IIIc) setzt eine Lymphonodektomie (in allen Fällen?) voraus.

Dabei ist nicht berücksichtigt, daß eine große Zahl der Patientinnen sehr adipös und alt ist, und daß das Risiko von Lymphknotenmetastasen gerade bei diesen sehr gering ist. Da es noch wesentlich mehr Probleme in der Definition der verschiedenen Stadien gibt, ist eine Periode des Übergangs und insbesondere ein Vergleich beider Staging-Modalitäten notwendig.

Tabelle 1: Endometrium-Karzinom, UFK Freiburg

Behandlungs zeitraum	OP außerhalb	Therapie UFK n	Alter (median)	Hysterektomie alle Stadien
1969-71	13%	260	63,8	36%
1974-76	34%	254	64,8	63%
1979-81	57%	153	67,3	79%
1984-86	47%	148	69,1	84%

Tabelle 2: Endometriumkarzinom, Stadieneinteilung FIGO Oktober 1988

Stadium		Differenzierung	
I	A	1/2/3	Tumor auf das Endometrium beschränkt
	B	1/2/3	Invasion bis 50% der Myometriumdicke
	C	1/2/3	Invasion über 50%
II	A	1/2/3	Tumor auf endozervikale Drüsen beschränkt
	B	1/2/3	Invasion des Stroma der Zervix
III	A	1/2/3	Befall der Uterus-Serosa und/oder Befall der Adnexe und/oder positive Peritonealzytologie
	B	1/2/3	Befall der Vagina
	C	1/2/3	Befall der pelvinen/paraaortalen Lymphknoten
IV	A	1/2/3	Invasion in die Blase und/oder Darmmukosa
	B	1/2/3	Fernmetastasen einschließlich intraabdominaler Metastasen und/oder Leistenlymphknoten

Beachte: Die Stadieneinteilung erfolgt ab jetzt postoperativ unter Berücksichtigung der Histologie und Zytologie. Primär bestrahlte Fälle werden klinisch eingestuft.

Tabelle 3: Endometrium-Karzinom*, postoperatives (chirurgisches) Stadium

		I	II	III	IV	alle	
praeop		0	3	0	2	0	5 (1%)
Stadium	I	256	22	12	8	298	(63%)
	II	33	54	12	5	104	(23%)
	III	1	3	22	12	38	(8%)
	IV	0	0	1	13	14	(3%)
alle		293	79	49	38	459*	
		(63,8%)	(17,2%)	(10,7%)	(8,3%)		

* eingeschlossen: 73 Fälle primär bestrahlt, 21 gemischte Müller-Tumoren, 3 Stromasarkome

Tabelle 4: Endometrium Karzinom*, 5-Jahresüberlebensrate

(Mo)	alte Stadieneinteilung präoperativ			neue Stadieneinteilung postoperativ		
	n > 5-Jahre		median (Mo)	n > 5-Jahre		median
Stadium I	297	69,8%	60,0+	293	74,0%	60,0+
Stadium II	104	63,1%	60,0+	79	57,7%	60,0+
Stadium III	38	23,5%	11,4	49	43,0%	45,9
Stadium IV	14	0%	14,8	38	8,2%	10,2

* eingeschlossen sind 73 primär bestrahlte Fälle

Mir erscheint es allein bedeutsam, die low-risk-Fälle, bei denen keine Lymphknotenmetastasen zu erwarten sind und bei denen damit eine Lymphonodektomie nur gefährlich ist, von high-risk-Fällen zu unterscheiden, bei denen die Lymphonodektomie für die Diagnose essentiell ist und vielleicht sogar für das Therapieergebnis Bedeutung hat.

2. Die Messung der Invasionstiefe in das Myometrium

Ein wichtiger Faktor für diese Entscheidung ist die Invasionstiefe im Myometrium. Die transabdominale Sonographie hat sich zwar für die Erkennung einer Zervixbeteiligung nicht bewährt, sie erlaubt aber die Messung der Invasionstiefe in das Myometrium. *Abdominale Sonographie* und *Kernspinresonanz* (NMR) ergeben gut vergleichbare Resultate [19,41]. Belloni u.a. [4] verglichen in 30 Fällen präoperative NMR-Messungen mit der histologischen Diagnose. Mit einem 1,5-T-Magnet- und der Spinechotechnik konnte in kontinuierlichen 4 mm auseinanderliegenden Schnitten in der Sagittalebene das Ausmaß der myometranen Invasion in 86%, und in 90% die Invasion in die Zervix richtig beurteilt werden. Auch Chen u.a. [11] sagten in 17 von 18 Fällen die nachfolgend histologisch festgestellte tiefe Invasion richtig voraus. Alle 3 Fälle mit Invasion in die Zervixwand und alle 6 Fälle mit ausgedehnter extrauteriner Ausbreitung wurden ebenfalls erkannt.

Etwa gleich gute Resultate, jedoch einfacher und billiger, sind mit der *vaginalen Sonographie* zu erzielen. Cacciatore u.a.[10] sagten die Invasionstiefe in 87% der Fälle (20 von 23) richtig voraus. In zwei Fällen war der Grad der Invasion tiefer als vorhergesagt und in einem Fall weniger tief als bei der vaginalen Sonographie gemessen wurde. Die abdominale Sonographie war nur in 78% der Fälle korrekt. Auch eine Beteiligung der Endozervix läßt sich mit der vaginalen Sonographie feststellen. Da eine Ovarialzyste über dem kleinen Becken bei der Vaginalsonographie übersehen wurde, empfehlen die Autoren zusätzlich immer eine abdominale Sonographie.

Für die endgültige Entscheidung zur Lymphonodektomie empfiehlt sich eine Betrachtung der Uteruswand während der Operation. Die makroskopische Betrachtung des frischen Gewebes erlaubt eine richtige Bestimmung der Invasionstiefe bei hochdifferenzierten Karzinomen in 87%, bei entdifferenzierten (G III) Karzinomen aber nur in 31% [18]. Die makroskopische Betrachtung des frischen Uterus wird mit zunehmendem Entdifferenzierungsgrad immer unsicherer. Fanning u.a.[15] überprüften die Aussagekraft einer Bestimmung der Invasionstiefe prospektiv an Schnellschnittpräparaten von 216 Fällen. Dazu wurden routinemäßig vier Schnitte durch die Uteruswand gelegt. Als tiefe myometrane Invasion galten mehr als 50% der Myometriumdicke. Die Richtigkeit der Vorhersage im positiven Sinn betrug 98%, im negativen Sinn 94%. Gestützt auf die Bestimmung der Invasionstiefe, einer Invasion der Zervix oder einer makroskopisch erkennbaren Invasion der Adnexe sowie bei allen Fällen, die im Abrasionsmaterial als G

III bezeichnet wurden, wurde eine paraaortale Lymphonodektomie vorgenommen. Von 216 Fällen im Stadium I waren dies 65 Fälle (32%). Bei diesen praeoperativ als Stadium I bezeichneten 65 fanden sich bei 16 (25%) paraaortale Lymphknotenmetastasen.

3. Folgerungen für das operative Vorgehen

Berücksichtigt man alle diese Daten, so sollte es möglich sein, low- und high-risk-Fälle prä- und intraoperativ zu unterscheiden. Handelt es sich um einen low-risk-Fall, definiert als Progesteronrezeptor mehr als 50 fmol, G I und G II, endometrioides Adenokarzinom, diploid und ohne Infiltration des äußeren Drittels des Myometriums, so empfehlen wir eine abdominale Hysterektomie unter Mitnahme beider Adnexe, eine sorgfältige Revision des Abdomens und eine Abtastung der Lymphknoten, aber *keine* Lymphonodektomie [31,32]. Handelt es sich dagegen um einen high-risk-Fall (Progesteronrezeptor weniger als 50 fmol, G III, seröser, hellzelliger, adenosquamöser oder sarkomatöser Typ, nicht-diploid, und infiltrierend in das äußere Drittel), so ist zumindest eine vollständige pelvine Lymphonodektomie indiziert.

Wenn sich bei diesem operativen Vorgehen Tumorgewebe außerhalb des Uterus findet, ist die Prognose sehr ungünstig. In diesen Fällen ist postoperativ eine adjuvante Therapie zu diskutieren.

E. Adjuvante postoperative Therapie

1. Strahlentherapie

Handelt es sich um einen low-risk-Fall oder um einen optimal operierten high-risk-Fall ohne Karzinom außerhalb des Uterus, sehen wir auf der Basis der Resultate der bekannten randomisierten Studie des Radium-Hospitals Oslo [1] keine Indikation für eine *perkutane Strahlentherapie* des kleinen Beckens. Im Falle einer low-risk-Situation besteht wegen der guten Prognose keine Indikation. Im Falle der high-risk-Situation halten wir eine Strahlentherapie wegen der in 12,5% beobachteten schweren Komplikationen [25] für gefährlich. Das gilt natürlich nicht für die high-risk-Fälle, bei denen keine optimale pelvine Lymphonodektomie durchgeführt worden ist.

Die *Kontaktbestrahlung des Scheidenstumpfes* mit Radium bzw. Iridium führten wir bisher in allen Fällen durch, da wir einzelne vaginale Rezidive bei low-risk-Fällen (G I, rezeptorpositiv, nicht infiltrierendes Karzinom) ohne postoperative Strahlentherapie der Vagina gesehen haben. Wir verwenden eine High-dose-rate 192-Iridium-After-Loading-Methode und bestrahlen 40 Gy in 4 Einzeldosen zu je 10 Gy im Abstand von mindestens 1 Woche. Bei dieser Bestrahlungstechnik haben wir dann, wenn keine perkutane Strahlentherapie zusätzlich vorgenommen worden ist, keine Fistel beobachtet.

Zum Thema der intravaginalen Kontaktbestrahlung haben Sorbe und Smeds [38] eine Studie an 404 operierten Stadium-I-Fällen des Endometriumkarzinoms vorgelegt. Alle Patientinnen wurden mit einer High-doserate After-Loading-Technik unter Verwendung einer 60 Co-Quelle (Cathetron) und einem zylindrischen Vaginalapplikator durchgeführt. Alle Patientinnen waren mit abdominaler Hysterektomie mit bilateraler Salpingo-Oophorektomie ohne Lymphknotensampling vorbehandelt.

Die Dosisrate betrug 0,5-1,0 Gy pro Minute in 1 cm Tiefe. Die Autoren verwandten 4 verschiedene Fraktionierungsschemata: 4x9 Gy, 5x6 Gy, 6x5 Gy und 6x4,5 Gy. Von den 404 Patientinnen entwickelten 15 (3,7%) ein Rezidiv. 0,7% der Patientinnen bekamen das Rezidiv in der Vagina (1 x im Scheidengewölbe und 2 x im distalen Drittel der Vagina), 1,7% in der Vagina und (oder) im Becken, 1,2% als Fernmetastasen und 0,7% regional und als Fernmetastasen. Zwei Drittel der Rezidive traten innerhalb von 2 Jahren auf. Eine statistische Analyse ergab, daß die myometrane Infiltration der zuverlässigste Prädiktor und die einzige signifikante Variable für die Wahrscheinlichkeit eines Rezidivs war. An Nebenwirkungen wurden in 16,3% Frühreaktionen an der Blase, in 19,6% Frühreaktionen am Darm, in 8,2% Spätreaktionen in der Blase und in 10,1% Spätreaktionen am Darm registriert. Die Spätreaktionen traten in 11,2% bei den 6x4,5 Gy Bestrahlten, und in 87,5% bei den 4x9,0 Gy Bestrahlten auf. In dieser letzteren Gruppe waren alle Reaktionen Grad II oder stärker. Von den Patientinnen, die noch sexuell aktiv waren (37,2%), klagten 66,2% nach der Bestrahlung über eine Dyspareunie verschiedenen Ausmaßes. Aus dieser exzellent dokumentierten Studie ergibt sich einerseits, daß bei einer Invasion des äußeren Drittels des Uterus eine Strahlentherapie der Vagina zu empfehlen und wahrscheinlich nötig ist, andererseits aber auch, daß man bei low-risk-Fällen wegen der doch unterschätzten Nebenwirkungen, auf eine routinemäßige Bestrahlung der Vagina verzichten sollte.

2. Adjuvante Hormontherapie

a. Adjuvante Gestagentherapie

Aufbauend auf Berichten über die erfolgreiche Behandlung rezidivierender Endometriumkarzinome mit Gestagenen mit einer Ansprechrate von über 30–40% in der früheren Literatur initiierte Kolstad 1975 eine Studie bei 1148 Patientinnen mit einem Endometriumkarzinom, die 1975–1982 in Oslo primär behandelt wurden [42]. Alle diese Patientinnen waren im klinischen Stadium I oder II, waren behandelt durch Hysterektomie und bilaterale Salpingo-Oophorektomie und in typischer Weise bestrahlt. Dabei hatten Patientinnen mit einer Infiltration der äußeren Hälfte des Myometriums oder mit Grad III-Tumoren eine externe pelvine Bestrahlung, alle anderen nur eine Bestrahlung des Scheidengewölbes mit Radium erhalten. Im Falle des Stadium-II waren die Patientinnen präoperativ mit intrakavitärem Radium vorbestrahlt worden. Verglichen mit einer (randomisierten) Kontrollgruppe von 531 Fällen erhielten 553 Fälle postoperativ eine Progestagenbehandlung. Die Behandlung begann 1–6 Wochen nach der Operation. Dabei erhielten die Patientinnen zunächst in 5 Tagen täglich 1,0 g Hydroxyprogesteroncapronat, später 2 x wöchentlich diese Dosis intramuskulär für insgesamt 1 Jahr. Nach einer medianen Beobachtungszeit von 72 Monaten und nach einer sorgfältigen klinischen und allgemeinen Untersuchung, einschließlich eines Interviews nach standardisiertem Fragebogen, ergab sich kein Unterschied in der Überlebenszeit der Patientinnen mit Progestagen und ohne. Auch bezüglich der Zahl der Patientinnen mit krebsbedingter Mortalität bestand kein Unterschied. Die Zahl der Todesfälle an interkurrenter Erkrankung war jedoch in der Progestagengruppe signifikant höher. Der Tod durch cardiovasculäre Erkrankung war in der Progestagengruppe innerhalb der ersten 2 Jahre tendenziell (p=0,07) höher. Lediglich die mediane Überlebenszeit der Patientinnen mit krebsbedingtem Tod war in der Progestagenbehandelten Gruppe länger als in der Kontrollgruppe. Dieser Unterschied war für die Subgruppen mit prognostisch ungünstigen Variablen (Stadium II, Infiltration der Serosa oder Gefäßeinbruch) ebenfalls signifikant. Ein Unterschied in der Rezidivrate fand sich jedoch nicht. Zusammenfassend ergibt sich aus dieser exzellenten Studie, daß bei low-risk-Fällen die adjuvante Gestagengabe vermehrt vaskulär bedingte Todesfälle zur Folge hat, während sich nur für high-risk-Patientinnen Nutzen und Schaden aufwiegen. Hier sind weitere Studien nötig. Diese Studien müssen aber die möglichen Nebenwirkungen der hochdosierten Progesteronbehandlung berücksichtigen.

Tabelle 5: Progesterontherapie bei rezidivierendem und metastasierendem Endometriumkarzinom (neuere Studien)

Präparat	Zahl der auswertbaren Fälle	CR und PR	Autor
Hydroxyprogesteroncapronat	114	16%	Piver et al. 1980
Megestrolazetat	88	11%	Podratz et al. 1985
Hydroxyprogesteronazetat	37	9%	
Medrogeston	26	12%	
Medroxyprogesteronazetat	347	17%	Thigpen et al. 1989
Megestrolazetat	20	20%	Pandya et al. 1989
Megestrolazetat + Tamoxifen	42	19%	

Tabelle 6: Endometriumkarzinom, Rezeptorstatus und Ansprechen auf eine Progesteronbehandlung, [13]

Rezeptorpositiv			Rezeptornegativ		
Zahl	Remission	%	Zahl	Remission	%
68	44	65%	111	11	9,9%

b. Gestagentherapie bei Rezidiv oder Metastasen

Die Progesteronbehandlung beim rezidivierenden und metastasierenden Endometriumkarzinom hat in jüngster Zeit ebenfalls neue Aspekte bekommen. Während man noch in den 60er und 70er Jahren von hohen Remissionsquoten schwärmte [7], hat sich heute Ernüchterung breit gemacht. Übereinstimmend ergibt sich, daß man bei rezidivierendem und metastasierendem Endometriumkarzinom bei Gestagentherapie eine Remissionsrate zwischen 10 und 20% erwarten darf (Tabelle 5). Besondere Beachtung verdient die große Studie der GOG, über die Thigpen u. Blessing [40] berichtet haben: Da bei 347 Patienten mit meßbarem Tumor unter einer Behandlung mit Medroxyprogesteronacetat (MPA) (3x50 mg/d p.o.) nur in 17% eine Remission aufgetreten war, hat man dies auf die zu niedrige Gestagendosis bezogen und eine zweite Studie (Studie 81) angeschlossen. Dabei wurde MPA in einer Dosis von 200 mg/d p.o. mit einer Dosis von 1000 mg/d p.o. in randomisierter Reihe verglichen. Von 236 auswertbaren Patientinnen zeigten auch hier nur 21% Remissionen. Dabei ergab sich, daß die höhere Dosierung keinen Vorteil brachte [40]. Es ist zu hoffen, daß die Remissionsrate höher liegt, wenn es sich um rezeptorpositive Karzinome handelt. Dies ergibt sich aus der Literaturübersicht von Deppe [13] (Tabelle 6).

c. LH-RH-Agonisten

Zur Behandlung Östrogen-Rezeptor positiver Metastasen bei jungen Patientinnen mit Mammakarzinomen werden heute LH-RH-Agonisten eingesetzt, da sie eine reversible Supression der Ovarien und damit eine direkte Verminderung der Östrogenspiegel zur Folge haben [37]. Unter solchen Bedingungen kann die Behandlung bei Endometriumkarzinomen mit LH-RH-Agonisten nicht indiziert sein, da sich die Patientinnen mit einem Endometriumkarzinom in der Mehrzahl aller Fälle in einer physiologischen postmenopausalen Ovarialinsuffizienz befinden und da die Entfernung der Ovarien im Rahmen der Primärtherapie fast immer erfolgt. Bei 52% der Mammakarzinomproben fanden jedoch Fekete u.a. [17] hochaffine LH-RH-Rezeptoren. Srkalovic u.a. [39] haben Rezeptoren für (D-Trp6)-luteinisierendes Releasing-Hormon auch in Endometriumkarzinomen entdeckt und charakterisiert. An Membranen von 31 Endometriumkarzinomproben bei Frauen zwischen 50 und 84 Jahren und von normalem Endometrium von 13 Frauen konnten die Autoren exakte Rezeptorbindungsstudien durchführen. Dabei fand sich eine spezifische Bindung von (125 J, D-Trp6)-LH-RH in Membranpräparationen von 77% (24 von 31) der Endometriumkarzinome und von 23% (3 von 13) der nicht-malignen Endometriumproben. Die Ligandenbindung entsprach der wie bei einem Peptidhormon. Natives LH-RH drängte das Analogon aus seiner Bindung und vice versa. Die Bindung war spezifisch. In denselben Proben wurden EGF-Rezeptoren in 85%, Östrogenrezeptoren in 86% und Progesteronrezeptoren in 90% gefunden. Die Daten von Srkalovic u.a. [39] ermutigen dazu, auch Endometriumkarzinompatientinnen mit LH-RH-Agonisten zu behandeln. Da die Rezeptoren im Karzinomgewebe stärker ausgebildet sind und häufiger vorkommen als im normalen Endometrium (im Gegensatz zu Progesteronrezeptoren), könnte dies besonders für entdifferenzierte Karzinome, also besonders für Rezidivfälle gelten. Klinische Erfahrungen liegen allerdings noch nicht vor.

3. Adjuvante Chemotherapie

Wie aufgezeigt, ist das Problem der Therapie beim Endometriumkarzinom die Behandlung der sogenannten high-risk-Fälle, speziell der mit extrauteriner Tumorausbreitung. Aus dem Jackson-Memorial-Hospital in Miami ist eine Untersuchung an 32 primär ausgedehnten Fällen bekannt [34]. Von den 22 Fällen des Stadiums III überlebten 6, von den 10 des Stadiums IV nur 1 mehr als 5 Jahre. Dabei zeigten die Patientinnen, die zur Operation eine Bestrahlung erhielten, ein besseres Ergebnis als die, die nur bestrahlt oder nur operiert worden waren. Die Hormontherapie brachte, wenn überhaupt, nur einen sehr geringen Benefit.

Wie zahlreiche vorausgehende Phase-II-Studien zur Chemotherapie des Endometriumkarzinoms ergeben haben, ist bis heute die Monotherapie mit Adriamycin, was die Remissionsrate anbetrifft, allen anderen Chemotherapien gleichwertig [32] (Tabelle 7). Von der GOG wurde deshalb eine randomisierte Studie an high-risk-Fällen des Endometriumkarzinoms mit einer adjuvanten Adriamycin-Gabe aktiviert. Das Ergebnis dieser Studie [34] wurde jetzt von Morrow u.a. [27] veröffentlicht. Alle Patientinnen waren nach der Operation bestrahlt worden (50 Gy kleines Becken, bei paraaortalen Metastasen zusätzlich 45 Gy paraaortal). Als »High risk« war eine Invasionstiefe von mehr als 50%, die histologisch bewiesene pelvine oder paraaortale Lymphknotenmetastasierung, die Ausdehnung auf die Zervix oder die Adnexe definiert. Von 181 auswertbaren Patientinnen erhielten 92 Adriamycin (45 mg/m^2) und 89 dienten als Kontrolle. Es ergab sich keine statistische Signifikanz der Überlebensraten in einem der beiden Arme und kein Unterschied in der Länge des progressionsfreien Intervalls. Die 5-Jahresüberlebensrate für Patientinnen mit tiefer myometraner Invasion, Zervixbeteiligung und (pelvinen) Lymphknotenmetastasen lag für beide Gruppen zwischen 63 und 70%, die für Patientinnen mit paraaortalen Metastasen bei 26%. Insgesamt kam es zu 5 therapiebedingten Todesfällen, 3 im zusätzlichen Chemotherapiearm, 2 im Kontrollarm mit Strahlentherapie allein. Das negative Ergebnis dieser Studie sollte nicht davon ablenken, daß ein wirksameres Zytostatikum zur Behandlung des Endometriumkarzinoms eine sehr wichtige Entdeckung wäre. Faßt man alle diese Ergebnisse zusammen, so ergibt sich, daß das Problem der Behandlung der high-risk-Fälle des Endometriumkarzinoms bis zum heutigen Tag ungelöst ist und daß eine effektive adjuvante Therapie nicht bekannt ist. So lange es keine wirksamen therapeutischen Modalitäten gibt, ist damit die postoperative Strahlenbehandlung bei allen Fällen, die Tumor außerhalb des Uterus aufweisen, trotz der bekannten Nebenwirkungen indiziert.

Tabelle 7: Endometriumkarzinom, Chemotherapie

		Zahl	CR+PR%
Monotherapie			
	Cyclophosphamid	33*	21%
	5-Fu	43*	23%
	Adriamycin	58*	34%
GOG 79	Adriamycin (60)	43	37%
GOG 81	CIS Platin (50)	25	4%
	Cis Platin (<200)	13	31%
Kombinationstherapie			
	ADM + Cis PI	29	52%
	ADM + Cis PI + Cyclo + Megest.	15	60%
	ADM + Cyclo + 5 Fu + Megace	20	75%
GOG 84	ADM + Cyclo + 5 Fu + Megace	>100	36,8%
	Melph + 5 Fu + Megace	26*	77%
GOG 84	Melph + 5 Fu + Megace	>100	36,8%
	ADM + Cis PI + Cyclo	26	60%

*Zusammenfassung mehrerer Studien

Literatur

1. Aalders J, Abeler V, Kolstad P, Onsrud U: Postoperative external irradiation and prognostic parameters in stage I endometrial carcinoma. Obstet. Gynecol. 56: 419-427, 1980
2. Annual Report on the results of treatment in gynecological cancer: Pettersson F, ed. Vol.XX, Stockholm 1988
3. Bauknecht T, Kohler M, Janz I, Pfleiderer A: The occurrence of epidermal Growth factor receptors and the characterization of EGF-like factors in human ovarian, endometrial, cervical and breast cancer. EGF receptors and factors in gynecological carcinomas. J. Cancer Res. Clin. Oncol. 115: 193-9, 1989

4. Belloni C, Vigano R, del Maschio A, Sironi S, Taccagni Gl, Vignali M: Magnetic resonance imaging in endometrial carcinoma staging. Gynecol. Oncol. 37: 172-7, 1990
5. Berchuck A, Soisson AP, Olt GJ, Soper JT, Clarke- Pearson DL, Bast RC Jr, McCarty KS Jr: Epidermal growth factor receptor expression in normal and malignant endometrium. Am J. Obstet. Gynecol. 161: 1247-52, 1989
6. Bokhman JV: Two pathogenetic types of endometrial carcinoma. Gynecol. Oncol. 15: 10-17, 1983
7. Bonte J: Results of adjuvant hormonotherapy in early endometrial carcinomas and of curative hormonotherapy in advanced or recurrent cancers by means of progestagens and antiestrogens. pp 250-255 in: Bolla M et al eds.: Endometrial cancers, Karger, Basel 1986
8. Borazjani G, Twiggs LB, Leung BS, Prem KA, Adcock LL, Carson LF: Prognostic significance of steroid receptors measured in primary metastatic and recurrent endometrial carcinoma. Am J. Obstet. Gynecol. 161: 1253-7, 1989
9. Britton LC, Wilson TO, Gaffey TA, Lieber MM, Wieand HS, Podratz KC: Flow cytometric DNA analysis of stage I endometrial carcinoma. Gynecol. Oncol. 34: 317-22, 1989
10. Cacciatore B, Lehtovirta P, Wahlstrom T, Ylanen K, Ylostalo P: Contribution of vaginal scanning to sonographic evaluation of endometrial cancer invasion. Acta Oncol. 28: 585-8, 1989
11. Chen SS, Rumancik WM, Spiegel G: Magnetic resonance imaging in stage I endometrial carcinoma. Obstet. Gynecol. 75: 274-7, 1990
12. Creasman WT, Soper JT, McCarty KS jr et al: Influence of cytoplasmic steroid receptor content on prognosis of early stage endometrial carcinoma. Amer. J. Obstet. Gynecol. 151: 922-32, 1985
13. Deppe G: Chemotherapy of gynecologic cancer. p. 158 Wiley-Liss, New York 1990
14. Einhorn N: The role of preoperative radiotherapy in the treatment of carcinoma of the endometrium. pp 53-61 in: Surwit EA and Alberts DS: Endometrial cancer. Kluwer Acad. Publ. Boston 1989
15. Fanning J, Tsukada Y, Piver MS: Intraoperative frozen section diagnosis of depth of myometrial invasion in endometrial adenocarcinoma. Gynecol. Oncol. 37: 47-50, 1990
16. Feichter GE, Höffken H, Hepp J, Haag D, Heberling D et al: DNA-flow-cytometric measurements on the normal, atrophic, hyperplastic and neoplastic human endometrium. Virchows Arch. 398: 53-65, 1982
17. Fekete M, Wittliff JL, Schally AV: Characteristics and distribution of receptors for (D-Top)-luteinizing-hormone, somatostatin, epidermal growth factor, and sex steroids in 500 biopsy samples of human breast cancer. J. Clin. Lab. Anal. 3: 137-147, 1989

18. Goff BA, Rice LW: Assessment of depth of myometrial invasion in endometrial adenocarcinoma. Gynecol. Oncol. 38: 46-48, 1990
19. Gordon AN, Fleischer AC, Dudley BS, Drolshagan LF, Kalemeris GC, Partain CL, Jones HW, Burnett LS: Preoperative assessment of myometrial invasion of endometrial adenocarcinoma by sonography and magnetic resonance imaging. Gynecol Oncol. 34: 175-9, 1989
20. Kauppila A, Kujansuu E, Vihko R: Cytosol estrogen and progestin receptors in endometrial carcinoma of patients treated with surgery, radiotherapy, and progestin, clinical correlates. Cancer 50: 2157-62, 1982
21. Kleine W, Fuchs A, de Gregorio G, Geyer H: Östrogen- und Progesteronrezeptoren beim Korpuskarzinom und ihre klinische Bedeutung. Geburtsh. u. Frauenheilk. 42: 884-7, 1982
22. Kleine W, Maier T, Geyer H, Pflederer A: Estrogen and Progesterone receptors in endometrial cancer and their prognostic relevance. Gynecol. Oncol. 38: 59-65, 1990
23. Koss LG, Schreiber K, Oberlander SG et al: Screening of asymptomatic women for endometrial cancer. Obstet. Gynecol. 57: 681-91, 1981
24. Lee KR, Scully RE: Complex endometrial hyperplasia and carcinoma in adolescents and young women 15 to 20 years of age. A report of 10 cases. Int. J. Gynecol. Pathol. 8: 201-13, 1989
25. Lewandowski G, Torrisi J, Potkul RK, Holloway RW, Popescu G, Whitfield G, Delgado G: Hysterectomy with extended surgical staging and radiotherapy versus hysterectomy alone and radiotherapy in stage I endometrial cancer: A comparison of complication rates. Gynecol. Oncol. 36: 401-4, 1990
26. Lindahl B, Alm P, Ferno M, Killander D, Langstrom E, Norgren A, Trope C: Prognostic value of steroid receptor concentration and flow cytometrical DNA measurements in stage I-II endometrial carcinoma. Acta Oncol. 28: 595-9, 1989
27. Morrow CP, Bundy BN, Homesley HD, Creasman WT, Hornback NB, Kurman R, Thipgen JT: Doxorubicin as an adjuvant following surgery and radiation therapy in patients with high-risk endometrial carcinoma, stage I and occult stage II: A gynecologic oncology group study. Gynecol. Oncol. 36: 166-71, 1990
28. Osmers R, Volksen M, Schauer A: Vaginosonography for early detection of endometrial carcinoma? Lancet, 335 (8705): 1569-71, 1990
29. Pfleiderer A, Kleine W: Risk factors of endometrial carcinoma. pp 12-21 in: Bolla M et al eds: Endometrial cancers, Karger, Basel 1986
30. Pfleiderer A, Kleine W, König P, Geyer H: Hormonal receptors in endometrial cancer. Analysis of clinical prognosis and risk factors. pp 35-46 in: Wolff JP, Scott JS eds: Hormones and sexual factors in human cancer aetiology. Elsevier SC. Publ., 1984

31. Pfleiderer A, Kleine W: Surgical methods and significance of different prognostic criteria. pp 119-128 in: Schulz KD et al eds: Endometrial cancer. W. Zuckschwerdt, München, 1986
32. Pfleiderer A: Der heutige Stand der Therapie des Korpuskarzinoms. pp 117-136 in: Künzel W u. Gips H eds: Gießener gynäkologische Fortbildung 1987, Springer Verlag Berlin, Heidelberg 1987
33. Pfleiderer A: Endometrial malignancy. Current opinion in Obstetrics and Gynecology Vol. 3, No. 1, February 1991 (in press)
34. Pliskow S, Penalver M, Averette HE: Stage III and IV endometrial carcinoma: A review of 41 cases. Gynecol. Oncol. 38: 210-215, 1990
35. Rosenberg P, Wingren S, Simonsen E, Stal O, Risberg B, Nordenskjold B: Flow cytometric measurements of DNA index and S-Phase on paraffin-embedded early stage endometrial cancer: An important prognostic indicator Gynecol. Oncol. 35: 50-4, 1989
36. Sainsburg JR, Farndon JR, Needham GK et al: Epidermal-growth-factor receptor status as predictor of early recurrence and of death from breast cancer. Lancet I, 364-6, 1985
37. Schally AV, Comaru-Schally AM, Redding TW: Antitumor effects of analogs of hypothalamic hormones in endocrine-dependent cancers. Proc. Soc. Exp. Biol. Med. 175: 259-281, 1984
38. Sorbe BG, Smeds AC: Postoperative vaginal irradiation with high dose rate afterloading technique in endometrial carcinoma stage I. Int. J. Radiat. Oncol. Biol. Phys. 18: 305-14, 1990
39. Srkalovic G, Wittliff JL, Schally AV: Detection and partial characterization of receptors for (D-TRP6)-luteinizing hormone-releasing hormone and epidermal growth factor in human endometrial carcinoma. Cancer Res. 50: 1841-6, 1990
40. Thigpen JT, Blessing JA: Progestin therapy for advanced or recurrent endometrial carcinoma: the gynecologic oncology group experience. Referat: Progestin Action and Progesteron Receptors in breast cancer, April 6-7, 1989, Washington DC, NCI, AG
41. Thorvinger B, Gudmundsson T, Horvat G, Forsberg L, Holtas S: Staging in local endometrial carcinoma. Assessment of magnetic resonance and ultrasound examinations. Acta Radiol. 30: 525-9, 1989
42. Vergote I, Kjorstad K, Abeler V, Kolstad P: A randomized trial of adjuvant progestagen in early endometrial cancer. Cancer 64: 1011-6, 1989
43. Wilson TO, Podratz KC, Gaffey TA, Malkasian GD Jr, O'Brien PC, Naessens JM: Evaluation of unfavorable histologic subtypes in endometrial adenocarcinoma. Am J Obstet. Gynecol. 162: 418-23, discussion 423-6, 1990

II. Prognosefaktoren

Histopathology of Endometrial Cancer

H. Fox

In this contribution the pathological features of endometrial adenocarcinoma that are of prognostic significance will be discussed.

A. Histological type

The histological classification of endometrial carcinomas is given in Table 1. Basically, the various types of neoplasm that can occur in the endometrium represent the multiple pathways of differentiation which are open to indifferent cells of Mullerian type. Thus, differentiation may be along endometrial, endocervical or tubal pathways to give, respectively, endometrioid, mucinous or serous papillary tumours.

The classification detailed in Table 1 is very similar to that currently recommended by the International Society of Gynecological Pathologists but differs slightly in regarding the adenosquamous carcinoma as a discrete entity rather than as a variant of an endometrioid adenocarcinoma.

The term »endometrioid adenocarcinoma« merits comment. The vast majority (85 per cent) of endometrial adenocarcinomas show some degree of endometrial differentiation and bear a resemblance, albeit an anarchic one, to normal proliferative endometrium; these are, therefore, »the usual type of endometrial adenocarcinoma«. A more succint alternative is, however, required for this unweildy phase and although the term »endometrioid adenocarcinoma« is not to everyones taste it is semantically, even pedantically, correct. Most endometrioid adenocarcinomas are reasonably well differentiated and easily recognisable as such but a minority are poorly differentiated and can only be recognised as being of endometrioid type if there is in some areas a tentative attempt at formation of endometrial-like glandular acini.

Table 1: Classification of endometrial carcinoma

1. Endometrioid adenocarcinoma
    Variants
    - with squamous metaplasia
    - papillary
    - secretory
    - ciliated
    - sertoliform
2. Adenosquamous carcinoma
3. Serous papillary adenocarcinoma
4. Clear cell adenocarcinoma
5. Mucinous adenocarcinoma
6. Squamous cell carcinoma
7. Undifferntiated carcinoma

Squamous metaplasia is very common in endometrioid adenocarcinomas and may be a conspicuous feature. There has been a tendency to class endometrioid neoplasms showing extensive squamous metaplasia as »adenoacanthomas« and these are regarded by some as a distinct entity having an unusually good prognosis. The criterion for recognition of such a tumour, i.e. the presence of »extensive« metaplasia is, however, ill-defined, imprecise and subjective. Further, it has now been clearly shown that endometrioid adenocarcinomas showing a striking degree of squamous metaplasia have a prognosis that does not differ significantly from that of endometrioid adenocarcinomas of similar grade showing no squamous metaplasia [2]. Hence there is little justification for considering the »adenoacanthoma« as a distinct nosological entity and this diagnostic term should be abandoned.

It is important to distinguish between the bland squamous metaplasia seen in many endometrioid adenocarcinomas and the malignant squamous epithelium which is present in an adenosquamous carcinoma of the endometrium. Tumours of this latter type account for about 5 per cent of endometrial neoplasms and contain both malignant glandular and malignant squamous components [1,11,15]. The glandular element is usually an endometrioid adenocarcinoma whilst the squamous component is clearly malignant and infiltrates the stroma in an invasive fashion. Adenosquamous carcinomas are aggressive neoplasms with a relatively poor prognosis [6].

An even more lethal neoplasm of the endometrium is the serous papillary adenocarcinoma [5,7,12,21]. These tumours are histologically identical to the serous papillary adenocarcinoma of the ovary, invade uterine lymphatic and vascular channels at an early stage in their evolutiom and are associated with a particularily gloomy prognosis [17]. The serous papillary adenocarcinoma has to be distinguished from a papillary endometrioid adenocarcinoma, a neoplasm whose prognosis does not differ from that of a non-papillary endometrioid adenocarcinoma [5].

The clear cell adenocarcinoma of the endometrium is identical histologically with clear cell neoplasms of the ovary and with those clear cell vaginal neoplasms developing in young girls exposed prenatally to di-ethyl stilboestrol [8,14,19]. This tumour also tends to invade lymphatic and vascular spaces at an early stage and has a very poor prognosis.

Mucinous adenocarcinomas of the endometrium, identical histologically to mucinous adenocarcinomas of the ovary and endocervical adenocarcinomas, have a prognosis similar to that of endometrioid adenocarcinomas of the same grade, this being generally very good [16].

B. Grading of endometrial tumours

Grading is probably only of prognostic value in endometrioid adenocarcinomas of the endometrium. It is certainly of little or no value in clear cell and serous papillary tumours [6].

Endometrial adenocarcinomas have traditionally been graded as well, moderately or poorly differentiated but this is a highly unsatisfactory grading system which is markedly subjective and in which there are no clearly defined boundaries between the various grades. The currently recommended grading system of the International Society of Gynecological Pathologists is:

Grade I: 5% or less of the tumour shows a solid growth pattern.
Grade II: Between 5 and 50% of the tumour is growing in a solid fashion.
Grade III: More than 50% of the tumour shows a solid growth pattern.

In making this grading solid sheets of metaplastic squamous epithelium are ignored. This grading system takes account only of growth pattern and neglects cytological features. Hence a codicil is added: Significant cytological atypia in Grade I or II tumours raises the grading by one grade.

C. Lymphatic space invasion

Lymphatic space involvement by tumour cells is an independent prognostic factor of considerable importance [10,20], being associated with markedly reduced survival rates. Even in Grade I, Stage 1 tumours the presence of lymphatic space invasion implies a relatively poor prognosis and the presence or absence of this finding should be an obligatory component of any pathological report on an endometrial neoplasm.

D. State of non-neoplastic endometrium

It is important to note and assess the state of any non-neoplastic endometrium which is present in an uterus harbouring an endometrial adenocarcinoma. It has been clearly shown that adenocarcinomas arising from a background of atypical endometrial hyperplasia are associated with a much higher 5 year survival rate than are those developing in an endometrium which is normally cycling, atrophic or shows a simple hyperplasia [3,18].

E. Depth of invasion

There is general agreement that the depth of myometrial invasion by adenocarcinomatous cells is of considerable prognostic significance [9], increasing depth of invasion being associated with increasing rates of recurrence and death. The reasons for this association are not entirely clear and it is also uncertain whether it is the distance from the endometrial-myometrial junction which is important or the distance from the serosa. Other points of issue are whether the depth of invasion should be stated in term of involvement of the outer third of the myometrium or the outer half and whether it would not be better to measure depth of invasion in terms of centimetres.

F. Assessment of cervical involvement

Although in general terms there is a reasonably good correlation between Stage and prognosis in cases of endometrial adenocarcinoma the quoted survival rates for Stage II cases vary rather widely [4]. This variability reflects the difficulties encountered in defining cervical involvement by an endometrial neoplasm.

The mere presence of tumour tissue within the endocervical canal does not, in itself, indicate cervical involvement and it is necessary to demonstrate histologically that the endometrial adenocarcinoma is actually invading the cervical stromal tissues. Replacement of endocervical epithelium by carcinomatous tissue, without invasion of the underlying stroma, is of much lesser prognostic importance [13].

References

1. Alberhasky RC, Connelly PJ, Christopherson WM (1982) Carcinoma of the endometrium. IV. Mixed adennosquamous carcinoma: a clinico-pathological study of 68 cases with long term follow up. Am J Clin Pathol 77: 655-664
2. Barrowclough H, Jaarsma KW (1980) Adenoacanthoma of the endometrium: a seperate entity or a histological curiosity? J Clin Pathol 33: 1064-1067
3. Beckner ME, Mori I, Silverberg SG (1985) Endometrial carcinoma: non-tumor factors in prognosis. Int J Gynecol Pathol 4: 131-145
4. Cavanagh D, Marsden DE, Ruffolo EH (1984) Carcinoma of the endometrium. In: Wynne RM (ed) Obsterics and gynecology annual. Appleton-Century Crofts, Norwalk, Conn. pp 212-260
5. Chen JL, Trost DC, Wilkinson EJ (1985) Endometrial papillary adenocarcinomas: two clinicopathological types. Int J Gynecol Pathol 4: 279-288
6. Christopherson WM (1986) The significance of the pathological findings in endometrial cancer. Clinics Obstet Gynaecol 13: 673-693
7. Christopherson WM, Alberhasky RC, Connelly PJ (1982a) Carcinoma of the endometrium. II. Papillary adenocarcinoma: a clinical-pathological study of 46 cases. Am J Clin Pathol 77: 534-540
8. Christopherson WM, Alberhasky RC, Connelly PJ (1982b) Carcinoma of the endometrium. I. A clinicopathologic study of clear cell carcinoma and secretory carcinoma. Cancer 69: 1511-1523
9. DiSaia PJ, Creasman WT (1986) Management of endometrial adenocarcinoma Stage I with surgical staging followed by tailored adjuvant radiation therapy. Clinics Obstet Gynaecol 13: 751-765
10. Hanson MB, van Nagell JR, Powell DE, Donaldson ES, Gallion H, Merhige M, Pavlik EJ (1985) The prognostic significance of lymph vascular invasion in Stage I endometrial cancer. Cancer 55: 1753-1757

11. Haqqani MT, Fox H (1976) Adenosquamous carcinoma of the endometrium. J Clin Pathol 29: 959-966
12. Hendrickson MR, Ross J, Eiffel P, Martinez A, Kempson RL (1982) Uterine papillary serous carcinoma: a highly malignant form of endometrial carcinoma. Am J Surg Pathol 6: 93-108
13. Kadar NRD, Kohorn EI, LiVolsi VA, Kapp DS (1982) Histologic variants of cervical involvement by endometrial carcinoma. Obstet Gynecol 59: 85-92
14. Kurman RJ, Scully RE (1976) Clear cell carcinoma of the endometrium: an analysis of 21 cases. Cancer 37: 872-882
15. Ng ABP, Reagan JW, Storaasli JP, Wentz WG (1973) Mixed adenosquamous carcinoma of the endometrium. Am J Clin Pathol 59: 765-781
16. Ross JC, Eiffel PJ, Cox RS, Kempson RL, Hendrickson MR (1983) Primary mucinous adenocarcinoma of the endometrium: a clinicopathologic and histochemical study. Am J Surg Pathol 7: 715-729
17. Silverberg SG (1984) New aspects of endometrial carcinoma. Clinics Obstet Gynaecol 11: 189-208
18. Silverberg SG (1988) Hyperplasia and carcinoma of the endometrium. Sem Diag Pathol 5: 135-153
19. Silverberg SG, DeGiogi LS (1975) Clear cell carcinoma of the endometrium: clinical, pathologic and ultrastructural findings. Cancer 1127-1140
20. Sivridis E, Buckley CH, Fox H (1987) The prognostic significance of lymphatic vascular space invasion in endometrial adenocarcinoma. Br J Obstet Gynaecol 94: 994-991
21. Walker AN, Mills SE (1982) Serous papillary carcinoma of the endometrium: a clinicopathologic study of 11 cases. Diag Gynecol Obstet 4: 261-267

Östrogen- und Progesteronrezeptoren beim Endometriumkarzinom

W. Kleine

Einleitung

Spezifische Steroidhormonrezeptoren vermitteln die Wirkung von Östrogenen und Progesteron am Endometrium im physiologischen Zyklus der geschlechtsreifen Frau. Seit mehr als 15 Jahren können Östrogen- und Progesteronrezeptoren im Zytoplasma und in der Kernfraktion von Endometriumzellen nachgewiesen werden [6,16,22]. Innerhalb des menstruellen Zyklus gibt es quantitative Unterschiede mit einem Gipfel von Östrogenrezeptoren zur Zyklusmitte, dem sich die maximale Konzentration der Progesteronrezeptoren unmittelbar anschließt. In Gewebsproben von prämalignen und malignen Veränderungen des Endometriums lassen sich ebenfalls Steroidhormonrezeptoren nachweisen – allerdings in geringerer Konzentration [5]. Es ergaben sich recht früh Hinweise auf eine Beziehung zwischen dem Steroidhormonrezeptorgehalt und der histologischen Differenzierung: je mehr das histologische Bild dem Ursprungsgewebe glich, desto häufiger ließen sich Steroidhormonrezeptoren nachweisen; entdifferenzierte Karzinome waren eher rezeptornegativ [13]. Die Steroidhormonrezeptoren beim Endometriumkarzinom scheinen auch mit anderen klinisch bekannten Prognosefaktoren wie beispielsweise dem Stadium oder der Infiltrationstiefe zu korrelieren. Schließlich ist es eine offene Frage, ob den Östrogen- oder den Progesteronrezeptoren eine eigene prognostische Bedeutung zuzurechnen ist.

Aus therapeutischer Sicht ist von Interesse, ob der Steroidhormonrezeptorgehalt bei Endometriumkarzinomen die Wirksamkeit einer Hormontherapie beeinflußt. Während beispielsweise beim Mammakarzinom der Östrogen- und Progesteronrezeptorgehalt eine wesentliche Entscheidungshilfe für die Wahl einer Chemo- oder Hormontherapie darstellt, sind die Erfahrungen beim Endometriumkarzinom relativ gering [3,17]. Dies mag auf die geringere Inzidenz und bessere Prognose des Endometriumkarzinoms gegenüber dem Mammakarzinom zurückzuführen sein.

Im folgenden sollen die Erfahrungen der Universitäts-Frauenklinik Freiburg mit der Bestimmung von Östrogen- und Progesteronrezeptoren bei malignen Tumoren des Endometriums dargestellt werden. Die Ergebnisse der biochemischen Bestimmung werden mit den histologischen Befunden und klinischen Daten korreliert, um schließlich den Rezeptorstatus als Prognosefaktor werten zu können.

Methodisches Vorgehen

Klinische Daten: Von 309 Patientinnen mit einem Endometriumkarzinom, die von 1979 bis 1987 in der Universitäts-Frauenklinik Freiburg behandelt worden waren, stand das Tumorgewebe für eine biochemische Rezeptoruntersuchung zur Verfügung. Die Stadieneinteilung der Patientinnen erfolgte entsprechend der FIGO-Klassifikation 1988 postoperativ aufgrund der histologisch gesicherten Ausdehnung des Karzinoms. Die Patientinnen im Stadium I wurden mit einer abdominalen Hysterektomie und einer Adnexexstirpation beidseits therapiert, postoperativ erhielten alle eine vaginale Kontaktbestrahlung und Patientinnen mit höherem Risiko zusätzlich eine externe Telekobaltbestrahlung des kleinen Beckens. Die Patientinnen im Stadium II und III wurden mit einer radikalen Hysterektomie nach Wertheim Meigs mit anschließender kombinierter Strahlentherapie behandelt. Auch im Stadium IV stand die Operation im Vordergrund mit der Zielsetzung, möglichst viel Tumorgewebe zu entfernen. Insbesondere bei verbliebenem Resttumor schloß sich eine Chemotherapie mit Adriamycin, Cisplatin und Cyclophosphamid an. Zusätzlich wurden Gestagene verabreicht. Die Behandlung der Patientinnen mit einem Rezidiv erfolgte individuell unter Berücksichtigung der Rezidivlokalisation und der vorangegangenen Primärtherapie. Im Vordergrund stand die lokale Excision mit anschließender Strahlentherapie und/oder die Gabe von Gestagenen. Patientinnen, die aufgrund ihres schlechten Allgemeinzustandes nicht stadiengerecht operiert werden konnten, eine primäre Strahlentherapie erhielten oder eine einfache vaginale Hysterektomie, werden bei der Auswertung hinsichtlich der Überlebenszeit nicht berücksichtigt.

Histologische Aufarbeitung des Gewebes: Der weitaus größte Teil der Gewebe wurde direkt aus den Hysterektomiepräparaten entnommen. Abrasionsmaterial von Patientinnen mit primärer Strahlentherapie oder lokale Biopsien bildeten die Ausnahme. Das Gewebe wurde in zwei spiegelbildliche Hälften geteilt und die eine Hälfte zur Steroidhormonrezeptorbestimmung bei minus 70 °C tiefgefroren. Der andere Teil gelangte zur üblichen histologischen Aufarbeitung mit Formalinfixierung und Paraffineinbettung. Alle Präparate wurden erneut durchgemustert und nach Adenokarzinomen, adenosquamösen Karzinomen, Klarzellkarzinomen und papillär serösen Karzinomen eingeteilt und der Differenzierungsgrad bestimmt. Aufgrund des makroskopischen Aspektes einbezogene endometriale Stromasarkome und Müller'sche Mischtumoren wurden registriert, gingen jedoch nicht in die Auswertung der Überlebenszeit mit ein.

Steroidhormonrezeptoranalyse: Das Gewebe für die Bestimmung der Östrogen- und Progesteronrezeptoren wurde nach der Dextran Coated Charcoal (DCC) - Methode aufgearbeitet und nach dem Scatchard Plot analysiert [8,10,19]. Die Qualitätssicherung war durch die Teilnahme an Ringversuchen gewährleistet, wie sie für die Rezeptorbestimmung beim Mammakarzinom bundesweit üblich ist. Die Grenze für rezeptorpositives Gewebe wurde bei 50 fmol/mg Zytosolprotein festgelegt. Dieser Wert liegt deutlich über der bei Mammakarzinomen üblichen Grenze und sollte dem Umstand Rechnung tragen, daß die Karzinomproben durch rezeptorpositives Myometrium »verunreinigt« sein können. Ein Grenzbereich von 50 fmol/mg wurde auch bereits von Ehrlich et al [3] angegeben, so daß wir uns seitdem auf diese Grenze beziehen, um eine Vergleichbarkeit zu gewährleisten.

Statistische Auswertung: Die Daten wurden mit Hilfe des Statistikprogrammes Siemens SPSS bearbeitet. Die Korrelation zwischen Steroidrezeptorgehalt, klinischen und histologischen Daten erfolgte mit Hilfe des Chi-Quadrattests, des Student-T-Tests oder des Pearson'schen Korrelationskoeffizienten. Die Überlebensdaten wurden nach der Methode von Bergson und Gage und die Differenzen der Überlebenszeiten nach Gehan und Wilcoxon analysiert. Für die Multivariationsanalyse diente das Cox-Regressionsmodell.

Ergebnisse

Von 309 malignen Tumoren des Endometrium ließen sich bei 164 (53%) Östrogen- und Progesteronrezeptoren von 50 und mehr fmol/mg Protein nachweisen. Demgegenüber waren 89 (29%) rezeptornegativ (Tabelle 1). Trennt man die malignen Tumoren des Endometrium nach ihren histologischen Typen, so wurde das histologische Bild von den Adenokarzinomen bestimmt. In 230 Fällen handelte es sich um sogenannte »endometrioide Adenokarzinome«. Fünf Gewebsproben enthielten Stromasarkome, die alle

Tabelle 1: Östrogen- und Progesteronrezeptoren bei malignen Endometriumtumoren

Rezeptorstatus	Maligne Endometriumtumoren	
ER+ / PR+	164	(53%)
ER+ / PR-	15	(5%)
ER- / PR+	41	(13%)
ER- / PR-	89	(29%)
	309	(100%)

ER+ = > 50 fmol/mg Protein / PR+ = > 50 fmol/mg Protein

Tabelle 2: Östrogen- und Progesteronrezeptoren bei unterschiedlichen histologischen Typen maligner Endometriumtumoren

Histologischer Typ		ER+ ER+	ER+ PR-	ER- PR+	ER- PR-
Adenokarzinom	n=230	137 (59%)	14 (6%)	33 (14%)	48 (21%)
Adenokanthom	n=20	12	-	2	6
Adenosquam. Karzinom	n=7	6	-	1	-
Klarzellkarzinom	n=3	2	-	-	1
Papill. Karzinom	n=21	5	1	3	12
Stromasarkom	n=5	-	-	-	5
Müller'scher Mischtumor	n=21	3	-	2	16
	n=309	165	15	41	88

ER+ = > 50 fmol/mg Protein / PR+ = > 50 fmol/mg Protein

rezeptornegativ waren. Von 21 malignen Müller'schen Mischtumoren waren 16 rezeptornegativ. Demgegenüber ließen sich bei den »reinen« Adenokarzinomen in 59% beide Rezeptoren nachweisen, 21% waren rezeptornegativ (vgl. Tabelle 2).

Tabelle 3: Anamnestische Daten von Patientinnen mit ER/PR positivem und negativem Endometriumkarzinom

Anamnestische Daten	ER+ und/oder PR+	ER- PR-
Menarche*	14,1 Jahre	14,5 Jahre
Menopause*	49,9 Jahre	49,5 Jahre
Nulliparae	21,0 %	22,0 %
Geburten*	2,4	2,5
Diabetes mel.	30,0 %	37,0 %
Hypertonie	68,0 %	65,0 %
Adipositas	62,0 %	36,0 %

* Durchschnitt
ER+ = > 50 fmol/mg Protein / PR+ = > 50 fmol/mg Protein

Die Analyse der anamnestischen Daten der Patientinnen zeigte keine Unterschiede zwischen Frauen mit einem rezeptorpositiven oder -negativen Endometriumkarzinom. Das durchschnittliche Alter bei Menarche und Menopause, die Parität und die typischen Risikofaktoren Diabetes mellitus und Hypertonie waren in beiden Gruppen gleich verteilt. Allerdings fällt auf, daß Patientinnen mit einem rezeptorpositiven Endometriumkarzinom doppelt so häufig übergewichtig waren als Patientinnen mit einem rezeptornegativen Karzinom (vgl. Tabelle 3)

Die Korrelation der beiden Hormonrezeptoren mit der Ausbreitung des Karzinoms ist in Tabelle 4 dargestellt. Im Stadium I ließen sich bei 70% der Endometriumkarzinome beide Rezeptoren nachweisen, während bei Rezidiven nur 19% rezeptorpositiv waren. Rezeptornegativ waren demgegenüber im Stadium I nur 10%, bei den Rezidiven allerdings 65%. Die zwischen dem Stadium I und den Rezidiven signifikante Korrelation war in den Stadien II, III und IV nur andeutungsweise zu erkennen.

Ein Zusammenhang mit dem histologischen Differenzierungsgrad konnte auch von uns in den untersuchten Gewebsproben beobachtet werden. Es wiesen 68% der hochdifferenzierten (Grad 1) Endometriumkarzinome und nur 25% der undifferenzierten (Grad 3) beide Rezeptoren auf; rezeptornegativ waren demgegenüber 9% der hochdifferenzierten und 55% der undifferenzierten Endometriumkarzinome (vgl. Tabelle 5).

Tabelle 4: Östrogen- und Progesteronrezeptoren in Bezug zum Stadium (postoperativ, FIGO 1988) beim Endometriumkarzinom

Rezeptorstatus	Stadium				
	I (n=138)	II (n=39)	III (n=36)	IV (n=32)	Rezidiv (n=38)
ER+ / PR+	96 (70%)	21 (54%)	17 (47%)	19 (59%)	8 (19%)
ER+ / PR-	9 (6%)	2 (5%)	2 (6%)	-	2 (5%)
ER- / PR+	19 (14%)	7 (18%)	4 (11%)	5 (16%)	4 (11%)
ER- / PR-	14 (10%)	9 (23%)	13 (38%)	8 (25%)	24 (65%)

ER+ = > 50 fmol/mg Protein / PR+ = > 50 fmol/mg Protein

Tabelle 5: Östrogen- und Progesteronrezeptoren in Bezug zum histologischen Differenzierungsgrad beim Endometriumkarzinom

Rezeptorstatus	Histologische Differenzierung		
	G1 (n=83)	G2 (n=138)	G3 (n=62)
ER+ / PR+	57 (68%)	90 (65%)	16 (25%)
ER+ / PR-	6 (7%)	8 (6%)	1 (2%)
ER- / PR+	13 (16%)	15 (11%)	11 (18%)
ER- / PR-	7 (9%)	25 (18%)	34 (55%)

ER+ = > 50 fmol/mg Protein / PR+ = > 50 fmol/mg Protein

Tabelle 6: Östrogen- und Progesteronrezeptoren im Bezug zur Infiltrationstiefe in das Myometrium

Rezeptorstatus	Infiltration des Myometriums		
	1/3 (n=87)	2/3 (n=53)	3/3 (n=75)
ER+ / PR+	54 (62%)	35 (66%)	39 (52%)
ER+ / PR-	6 (7%)	3 (6%)	3 (4%)
ER- / PR+	10 (11%)	8 (15%)	14 (19%)
ER- / PR-	17 (20%)	7 (13%)	19 (25%)

ER+ = > 50 fmol/mg Protein / PR+ = > 50 fmol/mg Protein

Tabelle 7: Östrogen- und Progesteronrezeptoren und mittlere Überlebenszeit von Patientinnen mit Endometriumkarzinom innerhalb der jeweiligen, postoperativen Stadien

Rezeptorstatus	Mittlere Überlebenszeit (in Monaten)				
	Stadium I*	Stadium II	Stadium III	Stadium IV	Rezidive
ER+/PR+	86% (n=86)	>60,0 (n=17)	>48,0 (n=11)	31,3 (n=14)	48,0 (n=8)
ER+/PR-	52% (n=9)	>54,0 (n=2)	- -	- -	9,0 (n=3)
ER-/PR+	88% (n=20)	>18,0 (n=5)	>36,0 (n=3)	>54,0 (n=3)	-
ER-/PR-	67% (n=14)	>60,0 (n=6)	>36,0 (n=9)	6,0 (n=4)	10,1 (n=20)
	p=0,0018	p=0,278	p=0,086	p=0,098	p=0,004

ER+ = > 50 fmol/mg Protein; PR+ = > 50 fmol/mg Protein
*Stadium I: % 5-Jahres-Überlebensrate

Die Infiltrationstiefe des Karzinoms in die Uteruswand gilt als ein weiterer Prognosefaktor. Einen Zusammenhang zwischen der Infiltrationstiefe eines Endometriumkarzinoms und seinem Rezeptorgehalt konnten wir nicht nachweisen. Bei gering infiltrierenden und bei tief infiltrierenden Karzinomen ließ sich eine annähernd gleiche Häufigkeit rezeptorpositiver und rezeptornegativer Karzinome nachweisen (vgl. Tabelle 6).

Der mögliche Einfluß des Steroidrezeptorgehalts von Endometriumkarzinomen auf die Überlebenszeit der Patientinnen ist in Tabelle 7 dargestellt. Die Auswertung bezieht sich allein auf die Frauen, die primär operiert worden sind, so daß die postoperativ getroffene Stadieneinteilung der aktuellen FIGO-Klassifikation entspricht. Patientinnen mit primärer Strahlentherapie oder unvollständiger Therapie gingen nicht in die Auswertung ein. Die Beobachtungszeit lag zwischen 6 Monaten und 9 Jahren, im Mittel bei 32 Monaten. Für Patientinnen im Stadium I ließ sich aufgrund der höheren Fallzahl und längerer Beobachtungsdauer die 5-Jahres Überlebensrate berechnen. Hier zeigte sich, daß die Patientinnen, in deren Endometriumkarzinom sich Östrogen- und Progesteronrezeptoren nachweisen ließen, eine bessere 5-Jahres Überlebenszeit aufwiesen als rezeptornegative Patientinnen. Bemerkenswert ist vor allem die Bedeutung des Progesteronrezeptorstatus: Patientinnen, die ausschließlich progesteron-rezeptorpositiv waren, hatten die gleich günstige Prognose wie Patientinnen mit beiden Rezeptoren. Der alleinige Nachweis des Östrogenrezeptors verbesserte die

Tabelle 8: Multivarianzanalyse verschiedener Prognosefaktoren beim Endometriumkarzinom (Cox-Regressions Modell)

Prognosefaktor		Relatives Risiko eß	
Stadium	(I,II-III,IV)	4,66	s.
PR (fmol/mg)	(>50-<50)	2,54	s.
Histologischer Differnzierungsgrad	(G1,G2-G3)	1,68	n.s.
ER (fmol/mg)	(>50-<50)	1,42	n.s.

(n.s. = nicht signifikant)

Prognose gegenüber rezeptornegativen Patientinnen nicht. In den Stadien II, III und IV ließen sich wahrscheinlich aufgrund der geringen Fallzahl keine signifikanten Unterschiede nachweisen. Allerdings zeigt sich bei Rezidiven wiederum die signifikant längere Überlebenszeit rezeptorpositiver Patientinnen.

Um die prognostische Bedeutung der Steroidhormonrezeptoren beim Endometriumkarzinom besser einschätzen zu können, wurde eine multivariate Analyse unter Einbeziehung der bekannten Prognosefaktoren »Stadium« und »histologischer Differenzierungsgrad« durchgeführt (vgl. Tabelle 8). Das Stadium erwies sich in unserem Kollektiv als der wichtigste prognostische Faktor beim Endometriumkarzinom. An zweiter Stelle rangierte der Progesteronrezeptor, während der histologische Differenzierungsgrad und der Östrogenrezeptor eine gewisse prognostische Bedeutung hatten, die allerdings kein Signifikanzniveau erreichte.

Diskussion

Im Gegensatz zum normalen Endometrium sind Östrogen- und Progesteronrezeptoren bei malignen Veränderungen nicht immer nachweisbar. Die Konzentration an Rezeptoren liegt in allen Fällen niedriger als im gesunden Gewebe [6,16]. In unserer Untersuchung wiesen knapp 60% aller Adenokarzinome des Endometrium beide Rezeptoren auf, 24% waren rezeptornegativ. Der Anteil rezeptorpositiver Karzinome liegt etwas niedriger als bei anderen Arbeitsgruppen. Hier zeigt sich das Problem, bei welcher Konzentration ein Karzinom als rezeptorpositiv gelten soll. Die einzelnen Arbeitsgruppen geben unterschiedliche Grenzwerte an, die z.b. für Östrogenrezeptoren zwischen 5 und 100 fmol/mg Protein und beim Progesteronrezeptor zwischen 10 und 50 fmol/mg Protein schwanken [2,11]. Die skandinavischen Arbeitsgruppen teilen das Gewebe in »rezeptorreich« und »rezeptorarm« ein mit einem Grenzwert von 30 fmol/mg Protein [7,21]. Die von uns bereits 1982 in Anlehnung an Ehrlich et al [3] gewählte Grenze von 50 fmol/mg Zytosolprotein findet sich so bestätigt und scheint biologisch sinnvoll zu sein. Sie sollte in jedem Fall deutlich höher als die Grenze beim Mammakarzinom gewählt werden, da beim Endometrium die Tumorzellen von rezeptorpositiven Zellen des Myometriums oder des Stromas umgeben sein können. Dies kann bei niedriger Gesamtkonzentration falsch positive Werte vortäuschen. Hier können heute immunhistochemische Untersuchungen die Rezeptoren in den einzelnen Zellen sichtbar machen und Probleme im Einzelfall klären [1,14,15]

Die Korrelation des Rezeptorstatus mit den anamnestischen Daten der Patientinnen zeigte, daß diese keinen Hinweis auf das Vorhandensein von Östrogen- oder Progesteronrezeptoren geben können. Auffallend ist lediglich die Beobachtung, daß adipöse Patientinnen häufiger ein rezeptorpositives Karzinom haben. Dies unterstreicht den Einfluß des Fettgewebes auf den Östrogenstoffwechsel in der Postmenopause [4,18]. Die fünf untersuchten endometrialen Stromasarkome und 16 von 21 Müller'schen Mischtumoren waren rezeptornegativ und stehen im Gegensatz zur Beobachtung von Soper et al [20], die bei zwei Stromasarkomen und 15 Müller'schen Mischtumoren häufiger Östrogen - und Progesteronrezeptoren nachweisen konnten. Bei den insgesamt kleinen Fallzahlen dieser Malignome ist es schwierig, weitere Rückschlüsse auf die Prognose zu ziehen. Hier sollten noch mehr Ergebnisse zusammengetragen werden.

Einen Zusammenhang zwischen dem Rezeptorenbesatz und der histologischen Differenzierung konnten auch wir bestätigen. Besser ausdifferenzierte Zellen eines Endometriumkarzinoms wiesen häufiger Rezeptoren auf als undifferenzierte Zellen. Auch bei umschriebener Ausbreitung des Karzinoms, im Stadium I, finden sich häufiger Rezeptoren als bei Rezidiven. Die sich daher aufdrängende Frage nach der prognostischen Bedeutung der Rezeptoren wurde am vorliegenden Kollektiv mit Hilfe einer Multivarianzanalyse beantwortet. Es zeigte sich, daß der Progesteronrezeptor ein signifikanter Prognosefaktor ist, der in seiner Wertigkeit direkt nach dem Stadium zu nennen ist. Demgegenüber hatte in unserem Kollektiv der Östrogenrezeptor keine prognostische Bedeutung. Diese Ergebnisse stehen im Widerspruch zu Mitteilungen von Martin et al [12], sie entsprechen aber wiederum den Ergebnissen von Richardson et al [17]. Eine genauere Analyse der Literatur zu diesem Thema wird von Kauppila im folgenden Kapitel dargelegt.

Für den Kliniker von besonderem Interesse ist die Frage, inwieweit der Hormonrezeptorstatus beim Endometriumkarzinom eine Entscheidungshilfe für die Wahl der Hormontherapie darstellt. Im Gegensatz zum Mammakarzinom liegen hier nur wenige Ergebnisse vor. An kleinen Fallzahlen konnte gezeigt werden, daß Patientinnen mit progesteronrezeptorpositiven Karzinomen in bis zu 89% auf eine Progesterontherapie ansprachen, während progesteronrezeptornegative nur in 17% von dieser Therapie profitierten [3,17]. Bei der retrospektiven Analyse des von uns dargestellten Kollektivs fand sich eine interessante Beobachtung: In der progesteronrezeptorpositiven Gruppe waren die Überlebensdaten zwischen Patientinnen mit und ohne Progesterontherapie gleich. Ebenso fanden sich in der progesteronrezeptornegativen Gruppe keine Unterschiede zwischen Patientinnen mit und ohne Gestagentherapie. Die Differenz der Überlebenszeit zwischen progesteronrezeptorpositiven und -negativen Patientinnen blieb allerdings erhalten [9]. Es stellt sich deshalb die Frage, ob die günstigen Überlebensdaten von Patientinnen mit einem progesteronrezeptorpositiven Endometriumkarzinom und einer Gestagentherapie auf den Progesteronrezeptorgehalt und die damit verbundenen biologischen Eigenschaften oder auf den Effekt des Gestagens zurückzuführen sind.

Literatur

1. Butwit-Novotny DA, McCarty KS, Cox EB, Soper JT, Mutsch DG, Creasman WT, Flowers JL, (1986) Immunhistochemical analyses of estrogen receptor in endometrial adenocarcinoma using a monoclonal antibody. Cancer Research 46: 5419-5425
2. Chambers JT, Mac Lusky N, Eisenfield A, Kohorn E, Lawrence R, Schwartz PE (1988) Estrogen and progestin receptor levels as prognosticator for survival in endometrial cancer. Gynecologic Oncology 31: 65-77
3. Ehrlich CE, Young PCM, Cleary RE (1981) Cytoplasmic progesterone and estradiol receptors in normal, hyperplastic, and carcinomatous endometria. Am J Obstet Gynecol 141: 539-546
4. Gambrell RD, Bagnell CA, Greenblatt RB (1983) Role of estrogens and progesterone in the etiology and prevention of endometrial cancer: Review. Am. J. Obstet. Gynecol. 146: 696-707

5. Hähnel R, Martin JD, Masters AM, Ratajczak T, Twaddle E (1979) Estrogen receptors and blood hormone levels in endometrial carcinoma. Gynecologic Oncology 8: 209-225
6. Jänne O, Kauppila A, Kontula K, Syrjäla P, Vihko R (1979) Female sex steroid receptors in normal hyperplastic and carcinomatous endometrium. The relationship to serum steroid hormones and gonadotropins and changes during medroxyprogesterone acetate administration. Int J Cancer 24: 542-554
7. Kaupilla AJI, Isotalo HE, Kivinen ST, Vihko RK (1986) Prediction of clinical outcome with estrogen and progestin receptor concentrations and their relationships to clinical and histopathological variables in endometrial cancer. Cancer Research 46: 5380-5384
8. Kleine W, Fuchs A, Gregorio G, Geyer A (1982) Östrogen- und Progesteronrezeptoren beim Korpuskarzinom und ihre klinische Bedeutung. Geburtshilfe und Frauenheilkunde 42: 884-887
9. Kleine W, Maier T, Geyer H, Pfleiderer A (1990) Estrogen and Progesterone Receptors in Endometrial Cancer and Their Prognostic Relevance. Gynecologic Oncology 38: 59-65
10. Korenman SG, Dukes BA (1970) Specific estrogen binding by the cytoplasm of hum breast carcinoma. J Clin Endocrinol Metab 30: 639-645
11. Liao BS, Twiggs LB, Leung BS, Yu WCY, Potish RA, Prem KA (1986) Cytoplasmic estrogen and progesterone receptors as prognostic parameters in primary endometrial carcinoma. Obstet Gynecol 67: 463-467
12. Martin JD, Hähnel R, McCartney AJ, Wooding TL (1983) The effect of estrogen receptor status on survival in patients with endometrial cancer. Am J Obstet Gynecol 147: 322-342
13. McCarty KS, Barton TK, Fetter BF, Creasman WT (1979) Correlation of estrogen and progesterone receptors with histologic differentiation in endometrial adenocarcinoma. Am J Pathol 96: 171-184
14. Mitze M, Jonat W, Brandle W, Kipke T, Stegner HE (1989) Vergleich immunhistologischer und biochemischer Östogenrezeptorbestimmungen an normalen hyperplastischen und neoplastischen Endometrien. Tumordiagn Ther 8/1: 1-6
15. Mutch DG, Soper JT, Budwit-Novotny DA, Cox EB, Creasman WT, McCarty KS (1987) Endometrial adenocarcinoma estrogen receptor content: Association of clinicopathologic features with immunohistochemical analysis compared with standard biochemical methods. Am J Obstet Gynecol 157: 924-931
16. Pollow K, Schmidt-Gollwitzer M, Nevinny-Stickel J (1977) Progesterone Receptors in Normal Human Endometrium and Endometrial Carcinoma. In: McGuire WL (HRSG) Progesterone Receptors in Normal and Neoplastic Tissues. Raven Press, New York, p 313-336

17. Richardson GS, Mac Laughlin DT (1986) The status of receptors in the management of endometrial cancer. Clin Obstet Gynecol 29: 628-637
18. Salmi T (1980) Endometrial carcinoma risk factors, with special reference to the use of oestrogens. Acta Endocrinologica Suppl. 233: 37-43
19. Scatchard G (1949) The attraction of proteins for small molecules and ions. Ann N Y Acad Sci 51: 660-672
20. Soper JT, McCarty KS, Hinshaw W, Creasman WT, Clarke-Pearson DL (1984) Cytoplasmic estrogen and progesterone receptor content of uterine sarcomas. Am J Obstet Gynecol 150: 342-348
21. Utaaker E, Iversen OE, Skaarland E (1987) The distributation and prognostic implications of steroid receptors in endometrial carcinomas. Gynecol Oncol 28: 89-100
22. Young PCM, Ehrlich CE, Cleary RE (1976) Progesterone binding in human endometrial carcinomas. Am J Obstet Gynecol 125: 353-360

Estrogen and Progestin Receptors in Relation to Conventional Prognosis Indicators in Endometrial Carcinomas

Antti Kauppila

Introduction

Determination of hormonal dependency by biochemical estrogen (ERC) and progestin receptor (PRC) assays have been found clinically beneficial in breast carcinoma [1,2]. ERC and PRC assays are being used e.g. in selecting breast carcinoma patients suitable for endocrine therapy. In endometrial carcinoma the clinical significance of ERC and PRC has remained unclear, despite receptor determinations, since the early years of the seventies in several centres. As in breast cancer, ERC and PRC assays seem, however, to be able to discriminate hormone sensitive tumors from those which are not hormine dependent [1-4]. The preliminary data from trials with a limited number of patients and short follow-up time about ten years ago suggested that they are clinically useful markers of the aggressivity of endometrial malignancies [5-6]. At present, several clinical studies with a sufficient number of patients with ERC and/or PRC assays and long follow-up time have been accomplished [4,7-18]. By reviewing the data from these studies, the present article is aimed at describing the available knowledge of ERC and PRC as prognosis indicators in endometrial carcinoma.

ERC and PRC in predicting prognosis

In 1983 Martin and co-workers [7] with a material of 87 patients suffering from clinical stage I-IV endometrial carcinoma showed that patients with ERC-positive tumors had a significantly better prognosis than patients with ERC-negative tumors. Thereafter results from 9 studies, each with more than 100 patients with stage I-II or I-IV disease, have confirmed that ERC and PRC are reliable indicators of prognosis (Table 1).

Table 1: Studies on the clinical value of estrogen (ERC) and/or progestin receptors (PRC) in predicting prognosis of endometrial carcinoma

Author, year (No of ref.)	Clinical stage	ERC No of pts	P	PRC No of pts	P
Studies with at least 100 patients					
Creasman et al. 1983 [8]	I-II	168	<.01	105	<.001
Kauppila et al. 1986 [9]	I	208	=.006	208	=.01
Lindahl et al. 1986 [10]	I-II	203	=.104	198	=.019
Ehrlich et al. 1988 [4]	I-IV	138	=.02	175	<.001
Chambers et al. 1988 [11]	I-II	187	=.003	187	=.0016
Palmer et al. 1988 [12]	I-IV	349	<.0000	349	=.0005
Ingram et al. 1989 [13]	I	Not evaluated		126	<.0001
Sutton et al. 1989 [14]	I-II	139	=.002	139	=.004
Kleine et al. 1989 [15]	I-IV	309	N.S.	309	Sign.
Studies with less than 100 patients					
Martin et al. 1983 [5]	I-IV	87	<.02	Not evaluated	
Utaaker et al. 1987 [16]	I-IV	71	N.S.	62	N.S.
Advanced disease					
Kauppila et al. 1986 [9]		25	=.045	25	N.S.
Borazjani et al. 1989 [17]		56	Sign.	56	Sign.

N.S. = not significant
Sign.= significant

ERC was an object of evaluation in 8 studies with a sufficient number of patients. Only in 2 of them [10,15] did the determination of ERC concentration fail to show any significant correlation of ERC to the prognosis. In the Swedish study [10] it might be due to methodological reasons since ERC was assayed with the isoelectric focusing method, whereas the other authors used the multiple-point dextran coated charcoal technique. There is not any explanation for the conflicting finding in the German study [15].

The importance of PRC as a prognosis indicator was evaluated in 9 studies. In each of them PRC was in significant correlation with the clinical outcome indicated with the disease-free survival or with the survival time. Also the size at the P-value in the statistical analysis of the importance of ERC and PRC as predictors of prognosis demonstrated PRC to be more precise than ERC in 6 of 8 studies. The combined use of ERC and PRC did not improve the accuracy of ERC alone or PRC alone in this respect [9].

There are also two studies in which the significance of ERC and PRC was evaluated in advanced endometrial carcinoma [9,17]. ERC was able to predict prognosis with a significant accuracy in both studies whereas PRC did so only in one of them [17].

Although in one Norwegian study with a limited number of patients both ERC and PRC were without significant importance as prognosticators [16], the other findings, reviewed above and in table 1, demonstrate that with the ERC and especially PRC determinations the patients can be classified into categories of low or high risk for recurrent disease. Receptor-positivity and/or receptor-richness indicate good prognostic prospects while the lack of receptors or receptor-poorness are reliable signs of increased risk for recurrent disease.

Multivariate analysis of clinical significance of steroid hormone receptors and conventional indicators of prognosis

Clinical staging, histopathologic grading of differentiation and depth of myometrial infiltration are the most important conventional disease-related indicators for prognosis in endometrial cancer. Together with such clinical risk indicators as the patient's age and her general condition they have played a dominant role in planning individual treatment strategies.

Table 2: Multivariate analysis of the significance of ERC and PRC as prognosis indicators in endometrial carcinoma

No Author year (No of ref)	Clin. stage	No of pts	Parameters evaluated	Significant parameters	P-value
Creasman et al. 1985 [8] (DFS) (Cut off values: 15 fmol/mg protein for ERC and PRC)	I-II	105	Cervical spread, Age, ERC, PRC, Extraut.metast. Extraut. met.	PRC Cervical spr. Age	<.0001 .0068 .0130 .0175
Palmer et al. 1988 [12] (Survival) (Different cut off values evaluated)	I-IV	349	Histol., Invas. Stage, Age, ERC10, ERC60 PRC10, PRC20 ERC70PRC30	Stage Age ERC70PRC30 (if withold ERC60)	
Chambers et al. (1988) [11] (Survival) (Different cut off values evaluated)	I-II	187	Grade, ERC PRC	-Continous variables: Grade only -Low, intemediate and high receptor classes: ERC only -Median values of receptors: PRC only	.045 .017 .005
Sutton et al. 1989 [14] (DFS) (Cut off values: 6 fmol/mg prot. for ERC and 50 fmol/mg prot. for PRC)	I-II	139	Age, Stage Grade, ERC PRC, Perit cytol., Adn. st., Invasion	Grade Perit. cytol PRC Age (cont.)	.0002 .0002 .004 .008
(Survival)				Age Grade Perit. cytol.	.003 .004 .04

Table 2 cont.

No Author year (No of ref)	Clin. stage	No of pts	Parameters evaluated	Significant parameters	P-value
Ingram et al. 1989 [13] (DFS) (Cut off values: 50 fmol/mg prot. for ERC and 100 fmol/mg prot. for PRC	I-IV	154	ERC, PRC, Perit., cytol., Grade, Horm. ther., Rad. ther., Cx invol. Adn. invol., Isthmic invol., Perit seeding, Invasion	PRC Cx involvement Perit. cytol.	<.0001 .0303 .08
Kleine et al. 1989 [15] (Survival) (Cut off values: 50 fmol/mg prot. for ERC and PRC)	I-IV	309	Stage, ERC PRC. Grade	Stage PRC	4.66* 2.54
Lindahl et al. 1989 [18] (DFS) (Cut off values: 400 fmol/mg DNA for ERC and 2000 fmol/mg DNA for PRC)	I-II	80	DNA, Grade ERC, Invasion DNA ploidy	DNA ploidy	.015
Borazjani et. al. 1989 [16] (Survival) (Cut off values: 2 fmol/mg prot. for ERC and ORC)	III-IV	56	Histology, Grade Site of met., ERC, PRC,	PRC Grade Site of met.	.0001 .0003 .03

In parentheses, indicator of clinical outcome, DFS=disease free survival, Cut off value of receptor concentration discriminating carcinomas to hormone dependent or not hormone dependent
*indicated as a relative risk

The observation that the findings in the ERC and PRC assays also correlate with prognosis had raised the question of their clinical importance and usefulness in relation to the conventional prognosis indicators in this disease.

Already Martin and co-workers observed that ERC provided information of prognosis which was additional to, and independent of, that provided by the histologic grade and myometrial penetration of the tumor [7]. This finding was first confirmed in a large study by Creasman and co-workers [8] and soon afterwards also by us [9]. In the study of the Creasman's group [8], the results in the ERC and PRC assays resulted in a more accurate prediction of prognosis than that provided by histopathologic grading of the tumor differentiation. On the contrary, in our study [9], the histopathologic grading was in better relation to the prognosis than the results in ERC and/or PRC assays. The discrepancy in these results may be methodological or due to differences in the subjective estimation of the grade of differentiation, or to differences in the sampling of the endometrial carcinoma tissue specimens for ERC and PRC assays.

In many recent studies [8,11-16,18] the significance of ERC and PRC as indicators of prognosis was evaluated in relation to several conventional clinical and histopathologic risk indicators mostly using Cox's stepwise multivariate analysis (Table 2). The investigation was carried out among patients with clinical stage I-IV diseases in 3 studies, clinical stage I or I-II disease only in 4 studies, and in advanced disease only in one study. The results from these studies are not directly comparable with each other since some of the parameters, e.g. the age of the patients or the receptor concentrations, were used as continuous variables or as variables grouped into few different size classes. As shown by Chambers and co-workers [11] the significance of the prognosis indicators may, to a certain extent, be dependent on the type by which the variables are presented. The results in the multivariate analysis were also dependent on the use of the survival time or the disease free survival (DFS) as an indicator of clinical outcome, as shown by Sutton and co-workers [14]. With DFS the significant prognosis indicators were histopathologic grade, peritoneal cytological finding, PRC and age, in this order. When DFS was replaced by survival, the age appeared to be the most important prognosticator and PRC lost its significance. The accentuated importance of age in the latter evaluation indirectly suggests that the defence mechanisms of the host against clinically manifest malignancy weakens with advancing age.

Table 3: Importance of different prognosis indicators of endometrial carcinoma evaluated in 8 different studies by stepwise multivariate analysis

Parameter	No of evaluations	No of significant findings	No of primary position
Age	3	3	0
Grade	6	3	2 (ref 11)
Stage	3	2	2
ERC	8	2	1 (ref 11)
PRC	7	6	4 (ref 11)
ERC/PRC	1	1	0
DNA ploidy	1	1	1
Site of met.	2	2	0
Cx involvement	2	2	0
Invasio	4	0	0
Perit.seeding or perit. cytol	3	1	0

Ref. 11, a study with 3 different evaluations

Certain conclusive remarks on the clinical significance of ERC and PRC and other indicators of prognosis can however be made. Also in the evaluations reviewed here, ERC and PRC proved potentially important prognosis indicators. PRC was a significant indicator of prognosis in 6 out of 7 evaluations (Table 3). Interestingly and importantly, PRC appeared to be the most precise prognosis indicator in 4 studies [8,11,13,16] whereas the histopathological grade had this position only in two evaluations [11,14]. ERC was weaker than PRC in most of the comparative evaluations, being of significant importance only in 2 out of 8 investigations. The significance of the clinical stage in relation to other risk indicators could be evaluated adequately only in 2 investigations with patients of all clinical stages [5,12]. Both studies revealed it as a most important indicator of prognosis.

It is worth underlining that the age of the patient was an independent and significant prognosis indicator in each of 3 evaluations made with female sex steroid hormone receptors in this malignancy. It may indicate that the age per se, in fact, has a modifying influence on the carcinogenetic and/or anticarcinogenetic processes in the human organism.

Desoxyribonucleic acid (DNA) measurements by flow cytometry have been the focus of increasing clinical interest during the last years [18-21]. In two studies comparing the importance of DNA ploidy and steroid hormone receptors as prognosis indicators, DNA ploidy appeared better than ERC or PRC [18,19]. In a recent study, DNA ploidy did, however, add no further prognostic information to that provided by clinical stage and myometrial infiltration [21]. Due to the conflicting observations, more data on prospective trials using fresh tissue specimens for DNA measurements are needed to show its clinical significance in endometrial cancer.

Conclusions

Recent clinical results from several studies have shown that the information provided by such traditional indicators of prognosis as the clinical stage of the disease and the age of the patient cannot be replaced by any modern predictors of the clinical course of the disease. Assessment of hormonal dependency by ERC and/or PRC measurement appeared to give information, which independent 19 of conventional risk indicators was in significant correlation with the aggressivity of the endometrial malignancy. Therefore ERC and, especially, PRC can be regarded clinically important prognosis indicators in this disease. As in breast carcinoma, they should be routineously determined in the clinical evaluation of each endometrial carcinoma patient.

References

1. Vihko R, Alanko A, Isomaa V, Kauppila A: The predictive value of steroid hormone receptor analysis in breast, endometrial and ovarian cancer. Med Oncol & Tumor Pharmacother 3: 197-210, 1986
2. Desombre ER, Holt JA, Herbst AL: Steroid receptors in breast, uterine and ovarian malignancy. Diagnostic and therapeutic applications. In Gynecol Endocrinol, eds JJ Gold, JB Josimovich, Plenum Publishing Corporation, pp 511-528, 1987
3. Kauppila A: Oestrogen and progestin receptors as prognostic indicators in endometrial cancer. A review of literature. Acta Oncol 28: 561-566, 1989
4. Ehrlich CE, Young PCM, Stehman FB, Sutton GP, Alford WM: Steroid receptors and clinical outcome in patients with adenocarcinoma of the endometrium. Am J Obstet Gynecol 158: 796- 807, 1988

5. Creasman WT, McCarty KS, Barton TK, McCarty KS Sr: Clinical correlates of estrogen- and progesterone-binding proteins in human endometrial adenocarcinoma. Obstet Gynecol 55: 363-370, 1980
6. Kauppila AJI, Isotalo H, Kujansuu E, Vihko R: Clinical significance of female sex steroid hormone receptors in endometrial carcinoma treated with conventional methods and medroxyprogesterone acetate. Excerpta Medica Intern Congr Series No 611. Proceedings of the International Symposium on Medroxyprogesterone acetate. pp 350-359, Excerpta Medica, Amsterdam, 1982
7. Martin JD, Hähnel R, McCartney AJ, Woodings TL: The effect of estrogen receptor status on survival in patients with endometrial cancer. Am J Obstet Gynecol 147: 322-324, 1983
8. Creasman WT, Soper JT, McCarty KS jr, McCarty KS Sr, Hinshaw W, Clarke-Peterson DL: Influence of cytoplasmic steroid receptor content on prognosis of early stage endometrial carcinoma. Am J Obstet Gynecol 151: 922-932, 1985
9. Kauppila AJI, Isotalo HE, Kivinen S, Vihko R: Prediction of clinical outcome with estrogen and progestin receptor concentrations and their relationships to clinical and histopathological variables in endometrial cancer. Cancer Res 46: 5380-5384, 1986
10. Lindahl B, Alm P, Fernö M, Grundsell H, Norgren A, Trope C: Relapse of endometrial cancer related to steroid receptor concentration, staging, hystol. grading and myometrial invasion. Anticancer Res 6: 1317-1320, 1986
11. Chambers JT, McLusky N, Eisenfield A, Kohorn EI, Lawrence R, Schwartz PE: Estrogen and progestin receptor levels as prognosticators for survival in endometrial carcinoma. Gynecol Oncol 31: 65-77, 1988
12. Palmer DC, Muir IM, Alexander AI, Cauchi M, Bennett RC, Quinn MA: The prognostic importance of steroid receptors in endometrial carcinoma. Obstet Gynecol 72: 388-393, 1988
13. Ingram SS, Rosenman J, Heath R, Morgan TM, Moore D, Varia M: The predictive value of progesterone receptor levels in endometrial cancer. Int J Rad Oncol Biol Phys 17: 21-27, 1989
14. Sutton GP, Geisler HE, Stehman FB, Young PCM, Kimes TM, Ehrlich CE: Features associated with survival and disease-free survival in early endometrial cancer. Am J Obstet Gynecol 160: 1385- 1393, 1989
15. Kleine W, Bergmann W, Geyer H, Pfleiderer H: Progesteronreceptoren beim Endometriumkarzinoma - ein entscheidender Prognosefaktor. Arch Gynecol Obstet 245: 1-4, 1989
16. Borazjani G, Twiggs LB, Leung BS, Prem KA, Adcock LL, Carson LF: Prognostic significance of steroid receptors measured in primary metastatic and recurrent endometrial carcinoma. Am J Obstet Gynecol 161: 1253-1257, 1989

17. Utaaker E, Iversen OE, Skaarland E: The distribution and prognostic implications of steroid receptors in endometrial carcinoma. Gynecol Oncol 28: 89-100, 1987
18. Lindahl B, Alm P, Fernö M, Killander D, Långström E, Norgren A, Trope C: Prognostic value of steroid receptor concentration and flow cytometrial DNA measurements in stage I-II endometrial carcinoma. Acta Oncol 28: 595-599, 1989
19. Iversen OE, Utaaker E and Skaarland E: DNA ploidy and steroid receptors as predictors of disease course in patients with endometrial carcinoma. Acta Obstet Gynecol Scand 67: 531 -537, 1988
20. Quillamor RM, Furlog JW, Hoschner JA, Wynn EM: Relative prognostic significance of DNA flow cytometry and histologic grading in endometrial carcinoma. Gynecol Obstet Invest 26: 332-337, 1988
21. Sorbe B, Risberg B, Frankendal B: DNA ploidy, morphometry, and nuclear grading as prognostic factors in endometrial carcinoma. Gynecol Oncol 38: 22-27, 1990.

Flow Cytometry in Invasive Endometrial Carcinoma

Claes Tropé, Janne Kaern, Bengt Lindahl, and Ignace Vergote

The frequency of endometrial carcinoma is increasing world-wide, and in most countries in Western Europe and the United States, it is now the most common gynecologic malignancy. In Norway, endometrial carcinoma is the second most common cancer of the female genital tract. Approximately 500 new cases are anticipated in 1991, and about 120 will die of endometrial carcinoma every year in our country. More individualized therapy is probably essential in improving the prognosis for these high-risk patients [1].

Tumor stage, degree of myometrial invasion, nuclear grade, histologic grade, and type have proved to be of prognostic value with regard to the risk of recurrence and long-term survival. The accuracy and reproducibility of these factors are not high enough [2].

During the past years the extensive application of automated methods for analytical cytology has resulted in a large quantity of data on ploidy disturbances in different types of human cancers. The main purpose has been to obtain additional parameters for the characterization of various types of malignancy in order to give more precise information on their biologic behaviour in addition to conventional histologic diagnostics. Flow cytometry provides a fast and precise method for determination of DNA ploidy and distribution of the cell cycle in tumors [3]. The major question concerning the clinical application of flow cytometry is the relation to prognosis, metastatic activity and sensitivity to treatment. Many studies have demonstrated that high DNA index values and a high proportion of S-phase cells are prognostic factors for survival (Table 1).

Normal human somatic cell in interfase contains 2 x 23 = 46 chromosomes, the number being referred to as diploid. Chromosome counts which are the multiples of 23 are referred to as euploid and a change in the number from a multiple of 23 is called aneuploidy. In a tumor, the most common number of chromosomes, the modal number, represents the cellines mainly propagating the tumor. The chromosome number of a tumor population could differ from that of a diploid one, some are in the tetraploid range and some in an intermediate position. Furthermore, aneuploidy could also be due to loss of chromosomes in diploid tumors. Since there is a close relationship between the number of chromosomes and cellular DNA content, the ploidy terms originally relating to the number of chromosomes have been applied to the DNA content for a tumor cell.

The DNA content of individual cells has been studied, using flow cytometry, by Lindahl et al 1987 in 112 histopathological normal endometrial tissues and in 222 endometrial adenocarcinomas. Aneuploid tumors often have a subpopulation of cells with a DNA index in the normal diploid region. This subpopulation is assumed to be composed of benign cells, but when counting the number of cells in this subpopulation in relation to the total number of cells in the tumor sample and comparing this to cytological findings, it was found that the majority of cells (70-100%) must be considered malignant. This so-called »normal« peak may thus not be suitable for defining the normal DNA index. Therefore the DNA index in 112 histopathological normal endometria was investigated and compared to the findings using the DNA index found in the diploid region in tumors with more than one cell population. The diploid DNA index was defined as the mean DNA index plus/minus two standard deviations. Using normal material gave more narrow limits (1,00±0,06 compared to 1,00±0,08 for malignant tumors). When ploidy aberrations were correlated to histopathology it was found that in well differentiated and moderately differentiated tumors 29% were aneuploid, respectively, but in poorly differentiated as many as 62% were aneuploid. The overall frequency of aneuploidy in endometrial cancer was 43% in this study. This is in the same range as in the studies of Iversen et al 1988 (30%, n=57), Feichter et al 1982 (27%, n=11), and Geisinger et al 1986 (33%, n=21). The relation with degree of differentiation was not examined in the latter studies. In the study of Lindahl et al 1987 there was no difference regarding the DNA index between stages I and II, but aneuploidy was more frequent in stage IV. The prognostic value of DNA ploidy using large scale flow cytometry analysis, was compared to staging according to FIGO, degree of differentiation, myometrial invasion and estradiol receptor concentrations. Three different ways of defining normal (diploid) DNA content were compared. The DNA index was defined as a modal DNA value of a cell population in relation to the modal DNA value of normal diploid cells. Thus, in a strict diploid cell population the DNA index was 1,00, while an aneuploid cell population had deviating DNA indices. Because of methodological errors (e.g. in sampling, storing, preparation and/or measurements) diploid tumors exhibit a variation in DNA indices around 1,00. In defining the normal DNA index, we compared the index found in normal endometria to the DNA index of the second peak of the tumors, which is almost always found in the diploid region of the tumors. In addition, this was compared to the number of populations, i.e. one population means diploidy and more than one population means aneuploidy. There seems to be a difference between the outcome using these different methods. There were fewer relapses among the diploid tumors correlated to normal endometria than among diploid tumors defined in the other way. In a Cox regression test the prognostic stability of the parameters investigated was compared. This analysis showed that the diploid DNA index limits, as calculated comparing with benign tissue, were better than diploid defined only as one population, and also much better than other known prognostic parameters such as degree of differentiation, myometrial invasion and estradiol receptor concentration. Our results were in agreement with Atkin 1976 and Moberger et al 1984. However, they used static cytophotometric methods, which do not have the same resolution. Iversen et al 1988 and Quillamor et al 1988 using the flow cytometric technique, have also come to the same conclusion as us, using the number of cell population to define aneuploidy. The death and recurrence rates were highest among patients with aneuploid or receptor poor tumors. We found almost the same risk of relapse using this definition of ploidy, but even with a higher number of patients no statistical significance was noted. Stendahl et al 1988 found in a prospective study of 185 women with endometrial carcinoma that patients with aneuploid tumors or tumors with high S-phase rates are at high risk for early recurrences. Our investigation was unable to verify the prognostic ability using the percentage of cells in S-phase, but found a very close relationship to the DNA index. This relationship means that all tumors with a high S-phase were aneuploid. Ploidy definition using the DNA index with limits of diploidy defined from normal endometrial tissue, proved to have a better prognostic ability than ploidy defined from the number of subpopulations, and also better than the percentage of cells in S-phase.

Table 1 shows that in 8 out of 10 studies the DNA index is an important prognostic tool in endometrial carcinoma. Iversen et al 1988, Lindahl et al 1987 and Britton et al 1989 found that it was the most important factor. This is in contrast with the retrospective study of Sorbe et al 1990 who found that DNA ploidy and nuclear morphometry did not add any significant prognostic information.

Our conclusion is that in future studies the DNA content of the tumor should be stated and not only the stage, grade, histological type and myometrial invasion. The ultimate goal is to find further possible prognostic information providing improved methods for choice of treatment.

Table 1: Endometrial Carcinoma - DNA ploidy

Authors	Year	No of Pts	Prognostic Value	Flow Cytometry	Comments
Atkin	1976	186	yes	-	
Geisinger et al	1986	21	no	+	
Lidahl et al	1987	222	yes	+	**
Iversen	1988	75	yes	+	**
Quillamor et al	1988	60*	yes	+	
stendahl et al	1988	185	yes	+	
Putten et al	1989	50*	yes	+	
Britton et al	1989	203*	yes	+	**
Moberger et al	1990	106*	yes	-	
Sorbe et al	1990	106*	no	+	

* = Paraffin embedded tumor material
** = The most important

References

1. Sorbe B., Risberg B., Frankendahl B.: DNA ploidy, morphometry and nuclear grade as prognostic factors in endometrial carcinoma. Gynecol Oncol 38: 22, 1990
2. Di Saia P.J., Creasman W.T., Boronow R.C., Lessing J.A.: Risk factors and recurrent patterns in stage I endometrial cancer. Amer J Obstet Gynecol 151: 1009, 1985
3. Iversen O.E.: Flow cytometric deoxyribunucleic acid index: A prognostic factor in endometrial carcinoma. Am J Obstet Gynecol 155: 770, 1986
4. Lindahl B., Alm O., Fernö M., Killander D., Långström E., Norgren A., Tropé C.: Prognostic value of flow cytometric DNA measurement in stage I-II endometrial carcinoma: Correlation with steroid receptor concentration, tumor myometrial invasion and degree of differentiation. Anticancer Research 7: 791, 1987
5. Iversen O.E., Utaker E, Skaarland E.: DNA ploidy and steroid receptors as predictors of disease course in patients with endometrial carcinoma. Acta Obstet Gynecol Scand 67: 531, 1988

6. Geisinger K.R., Homesley H.D., Torgan T.M., Kute T.E., Marshall R.B.: Endometrial adenocarcinoma: A multiparameter clinico pathological analysis including the DNA profile and the sex steroid hormone receptors. Cancer 58: 1518, 1986
7. Atkin N.: Prognostic significance of ploidy level in human tumors I carcinoma of the uterus. J Natl Cancer Inst 56: 909, 1976
8. Moberger B., Auer G., Forslund G., Mogerger G.: The prognostic significance in DNA measurements in endometrial carcinoma. Cytometry 5: 430, 1984
9. Quillamor R.M., Furlong S.K., Hoschner J.A., Wynn R.M.: Relative prognostic significance of DNA flow cytometry and histologic grading in endometrial carcinoma. Gynecol Obstet Invest 26: 332, 1988
10. Stendahl U., Wagenius G., Strang P., Tribukait B.: Flow cytometry in invasive endometrial carcinoma. Correlation between DNA content, S-phase rate and clinical parameters. In Vivo 2: 123, 1988
11. Britton L.C., Wilson T.O., Gaffey T.A., Lieber M.M., Wieland H.S., Podratz K.C.: Flow cytometric DNA analysis of stage I endometrial carcinoma. Gynecol Oncol 34: 317, 1989

Oncogenes in Endometrial Cancer: A Review of Information

Ernest I. Kohorn, Barry M. Kacinski

The intense and productive study of oncogenes of the past decade was stimulated by the realization that genes concerned with normal growth regulation are phylogenitically very similar to the viral genes long known to be associated with cancer induction in avian and rodent cancers such as the Rous sarcoma or the Bittner breast cancer of mice. The studies were made possible by advances in technology for the study of DNA, RNA and nucleoprotein physiology. Viral transforming genes are called viral oncogenes (v-onc). DNA sequences that exist in normal tissue are conserved in evolution from species as separate as yeast to mammals. These genes are homologous to the viral oncogenes and are called cellular oncogenes (c-onc). They regulate normal cellular proliferation and in the process of carcinogenesis are changed in detail of structure or in the amount of gene produced either by physical or chemical agents or, in human cancer, by yet unknown primary causative agents.

Presently, our knowledge of the changes in genes associated with human neoplasia is fragmentary, but the details of the inter-relationship and of function of the various oncogenes is gradually being filled in. Different cancers have different overexpression of some oncogenes. The oncogenes fall into several general classes; nucleoproteins, nucleotide binding proteins, growth factors and growth factor receptors. Table 1 sets out the functional association of some of the oncogenes and Figure 1 shows the site of the genes in the cell. Oncogenes are named usually from their viral gene counterpart. The oncogenes myc, fos, myb, and the cellular gene P53 code for proteins present in the nuclei of normal cells. c-myc, c-fos, and c-myb are expressed significantly in the early embryo and transiently in cells exposed to mitogens. P53 is present in normal cells as a short-lived phosphoprotein. The ras family of genes (ha-ras, ki-ras and n-ras) code for guanosine nucleotide binding proteins, related to the G-protein intracellular messengers. These genes also are expressed at high levels during embryogenesis and at low levels in non proliferating somatic cells.

Table 1: Oncogene probes used in in situ hybridization studies

Nuclear protein oncogenes

c-myc
n-myc
l-myc
fos
myb
P53

Guanosine triphosphate binding protein (second messenger) oncogenes

k-ras, h-ras, n-ras

Growth factor oncogenes

Platelet derived growth factor A chain
Platelet derived growth factor B chain (=sis)

Growth factor receptors and tyrosine protein kinase oncogenes

erb-B1 (epidermal growth factor receptor)
erb-B2 = neu
fes
fms (colony stimulating factor receptor)
ros (? insulin like growth factor receptor)
krk
erb-A (T3 receptor)

A further significant group of (onco)genes are responsible for growth factors. The sis oncogene codes for the ß-chain of platelet derived growth factor. hst and int-2 encode a gene for a peptide hormone related to fibroblast growth factor. Growth factor oncogenes that code for protein kinases are src, erb B1, erb B2/neu, fms, ros, kit and the receptor for platelet derived growth factor. The protein products of these genes contain domains for protein kinase activity linked to domains for membrane association that extend outside the cell to bind peptide hormone ligands. These tyrosine kinases have functions in normal cellular metabolism and it is an alteration in their structure or their excess expression that will make cells sensitive to mitogens.

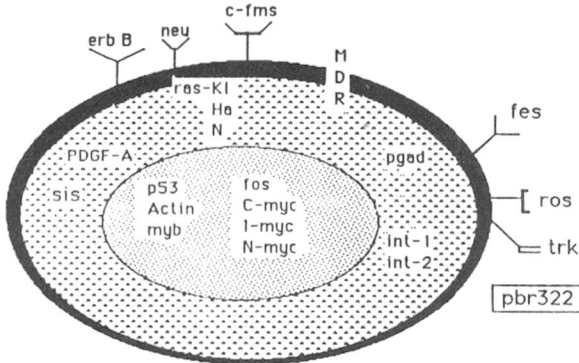

Figure 1: Schematic Representation of Oncogenes in Cell

Oncogenes and cancer induction

Oncogenes, that is regulatory genes, are usually under strict control and their expression is limited to defined times in cell regulation and cell growth. Oncogenes must be activated before they can participate to initiate or induce cancer. Activation occurs by the following mechanisms:

1. Overexpression by acquisition of an active promotor or following amplification of their DNA sequences.

2. Overtranscription and overexpression by an enhancer sequence.

3. Activation by mutational events modifying the structure and function of their protein products resulting in a neoplastic phenotype.

1 und 2 result in the overproduction of messenger RNA while 3 is associated with overexpression of a mutant gene or gene product. For the development of neoplasia the expression of more than one oncogene is necessary suggesting that a stepwise mechanism of oncogene activation is associated with the development of spontaneous cancer.

Techniques used for the study of oncogene expression [1]

Nucleic acid hybridization

This now well-established technique requires radioactive or chemically labeled »probe« DNA or RNA, the test nucleic acid to be tested for sequence homology and a means of detecting »hybridization« of the labeled probe to single stranded nucleic acids with sequence homology to the probe. DNA electrophoresis and Southern blotting allows the characterization of the DNA sequences from the tissue specimens of cell lines and shows gross rearrangement or duplication in sequence. Northern blotting and RNA electrophoresis or total cellular or total messenger RNA from tumor cell lines or from homogenous tumors permits the determination of increased levels of abnormal oncogene complimentary transcripts. However, as RNA is very labile and speedily degradable such specimens need to be immediately flash frozen in liquid nitrogen. In tumors with much stroma the level of RNA expression may be underestimated.

In situ hybridization

Biopsy specimens are immediately fixed and processed for paraffin embedding. Six micron sections are then prepared for incubation with specific single stranded radioactive ^{35}S probes of specific oncogenes. Following exposure and development, grain counting is performed on hematoxylin and eosin stained sections using an Olympus Corporation Cue2 VISION Image Analysis System. High power examination allows determination of the precise tissue examined for grain counting. Counts are compared to non-specific probe counts. The results are expressed as hybridized probe molecules per cubic micron of tissue.

Immunochemical methods

Western blotting is particularly useful in detecting oncogene antigen expression in non-radioactively labeled specimens. Non-specific cross reactivity causes problems. Immunohistochemical staining can localize oncogene antigens at a cellular level more precisely than is usually feasible by in situ hybridization methods. However, quantitation is difficult. The method is useful for formalin-fixed embedded tissue from archival blocks.

Oncogenes in endometrial cancer

At Yale, our initial search for oncogenes in human neoplasia began with hydatidiform mole, but soon ovarian, endometrial and breast cancer were also being explored as tissue specimens for these neoplasms were so much more frequently available. Our efforts concentrated on identifying the site of oncogene messenger RNA expression in the tissue and it became apparent early that the RNA was most frequently expressed in the neoplastic epithelial cells and very little in the stroma. This method of in situ hybridization allowed for precise localization of the oncogene and quantitation was achieved by a technique of computer grain counting developed by Dr. Kacinski. Gel electrophoresis at that stage was used mainly to confirm the grain counting results, but Southern blotting for DNA und Northern blotting for RNA became more important as the research used tissue culture of established cell lines more frequently. The initial search using 21 oncogene probes in endometrial cancer demonstrated the overexpression of fms, fos, c-myc and myb oncogenes in tissue samples [2]. Statistical analysis showed that only the overexpression of fms oncogene correlated at a very high level of statistical significance with the clinical parameters of high tumor grade and tumor invasiveness into the myometrium. Similar results were obtained with ovarian cancer [3]. With ovarian cancer cell lines grown in defined media on the surface of processed human amnion, cell invasion was demonstrated in the presence of fms protein product, CMF-1 [4]. CMF-1 was known to be a hemopoietic and specifically a macrophage growth factor and its presence in association with human epithelial cancer was somewhat unexpected [5].

To complement the initial finding of excess of fms oncogene in endometrial tissue, immunohistologic staining was performed on malignant and benign endometrial tissue. Using an anti-human CSF-1 antibody, 21 of 24 specimens of carcinomas and 4 of 11 benign lesions showed significant staining [6]. Immunological staining using the antibody to fms (CSF-1 receptor) antigen, showed positive staining of epithelial elements and of stromal macrophages in all 24 carcinomas and 3 of 11 benign endometrial lesions [6]. The 3 benign tissues were secretory phase endometrium.

c-fms (CSF-1 receptor gene) was demonstrated in the cultured endometrial carcinoma cell lines by Northern blots of total RNA [6]. By use of anti-fms antiserum, fms-antigen was demonstrable in endometrial cancer cell lines by Western blotting [6].

These data show that CSF-1 receptor gene is expressed *in vivo* in cancer cell lines and *in vitro* in tissue specimens of endometrial cancer similar to the findings in ovarian cancer [7]. CSF-1 receptor is also produced by tissue macrophages and by choriocarcinoma cell lines [5]. It is suggested that CSF-1 and its receptor may play a significant role in endometrial cancer physiology by stimulating tumor cell proliferation and promoting tumor cell invasion into the endometrial stroma and the myometrium in a manner similar to that which occurs with CSF-1 and its receptor with activated macrophages and implanting trophoblast [5]. This ligand activation may be paracrine or even autocrine.

Examination of serum specimens from patients with active or recurrent endometrial cancer by radioimmunoassay has demonstrated significantly elevated levels of CSF-1 [6,7]. This finding provides a new tumor marker for use in patients with endometrial cancer and as in ovarian cancer it is significant that serum levels of CSF-1 may be elevated in some patients at a time when CA-125 levels are normal. It would appear that the 2 tests may complement each other.

The fact that high levels of CSF-1 in the serum of endometrial cancer patients could promote the ligand activation of the epithelial cell CSF-1 receptor may be of biologic significance as this may further cell proliferation and cell invasion in the tumor [6].

The present state of knowledge of oncogene activation in endometrial cancer is that c-fos, c-myc and c-myb oncogenes are expressed in concordance with the cell proliferation present. c-fms, its product CSF-1 and its receptor have been found to be associated with mitotic and invasive characteristics in endometrial cancer. The immediate benefit in patient management is the availability of a new tumor marker, as CSF-1 may be measured in peripheral blood specimens from patients. The exploitation of this knowledge for therapy will require further research.

This research has been directed by Dr. Barry M. Kacinski and has been significantly helped by the following individuals:

Basic Science Research: Barry M. Kacinski, E. Richard Stanley[*], Larry Rohrschneider[**], Victoria Rothwell[**]

Yale University
[*] Albert Einstein College of Medicine
[**] Fred Hutchinson Cancer Center, Seattle

Pathologists: Darryl C. Carter, Khush Mittal

Gynecologists: Setsuko K. Chambers, Joseph T. Chambers, Ernest I. Kohorn, Peter E. Schwartz

Laboratory Staff: Kimberly A. Scata, Mary H. Pirro, David H-Y Chang, Josephine T. Nguyen

References

1. Ying LD, Kacinski BM, Carter D: Oncogene Structure, Function and Expression in Breast Cancer. Semin in Diagn Pathol 6: 110-125, 1989
2. Kacinski BM, Carter D, Mittal K, Kohorn EI, Bloodgood RS, Donahue J, Donofrio L, Edwards R, Schwartz PE, Chambers JT, Chambers SK: High Level Expression of fms Proto-Oncogene mRNA is Observed in Clinically Aggressive Human Endometrial Adenocarcinomas. Int J Radiat Oncol Biol Phys 15: 823-829, 1988
3. Kacinski BM; Carter D, Kohorn EI, Mittal K, Bloodgood RS, Donahue J, Kramer CA, Fischer D, Edwards R, Chambers SK, Chambers JT, Schwartz PE: Oncogene Expression *in Vivo* by Ovarian Adenocarcinomas and Mixed-Mullerian Tumors. Yale J Biol Med 62: 379-392, 1989
4. Foellmer HG, Oemar BS, Kohorn EI, Kacinski BM: Influence of Hemopoietic Growth Factors on Ovarian and Endometrial Tumor Cell Invasion. 4th Int Congress of Cell Biol, August 1988
5. Kacinski BM, Carter D, Mittal K, Yee LD, Scata KA, Donofrio L, Chambers SK, Wang KI, Yang-Feng T: Ovarian Adenocarcinomas Express fms-Complementary Transcripts and fms Antigen, Often with Coexpression of CSF-1. Am J Pathol 137: 135-147, 1990
6. Kacinski BM, Chambers SK, Stanley ER, Carter DC, Tseng P, Scata KA, Chang DHY, Pirro MH, Nguyen JT, Ariza A, Rohrschneider LR, Rothwell V: The Cytokine CSF-1 (M-CSF) Expressed by Endometrial Carcinomas *in vivo* and *in vitro* May also be a Circulating Tumor Marker of Neoplastic Disease Activity in Endometrial Carcinoma Patients. In Press, Int J Radiat Oncol Biol Phys, September 1990
7. Kacinski BM, Bloodgood RS, Schwartz PE, Carter D, Stanley ER: Macrophage Colony-stimulating Factor is Produced by Human Ovarian and Endometrial Adenocarcinoma-derived Cell Lines and is Present at Abnormally High Levels in the Plasma of Ovarian Carcinoma Patients with Active Disease. Cancer Cells 7: 333-339, Cold Spring Harbor Press, 1989

EGF Receptor (EGF-R) Analysis in Endometrial Carcinomas

Thomas Bauknecht

Introduction

A better understanding of cell growth and differentiation began with the detection of the proto-oncogenes [1]. In the process of tumor development and progression a modification of the structure and the function of these genes probably take place which are detected molecular-chemically as activated oncogenes [2].

The epidermal growth factor receptor (EGF-R), which is the product of the c-erb B1 proto-oncogene [3], enables cells to undergo DNA synthesis in response to either of the known physiologic EGF-R ligands, EGF and TGFa [4,5,6]. Abnormalities of the EGF-R gene especially an increased number of apparently a normal EGF-R have been described for breast [7], ovarian [8,9,10], squamous cell [11], gastro-intestinal carcinomas [12], and other tumors. For some of these tumors the EGF-R status seems to fulfill the criteria of an independent prognostic factor [7]. Another reason for uncontrolled proliferation is the inappropiate expression and production of growth factors such as TGFa [6]. It is believed that the aggressive behavior in terms of tumor progression is influenced by the growth properties of tumors which may be stimulated by the autonomous growth factor production of tumors in an autocrine or paracrine manner [6,9,10,13].

The endometrial carcinoma is one of the most common malignancy of the female genital tract [14] and its prognosis depends on its growth and invasion properties. Clinically, the tumor stage, the histological subtype, the grade of differentiation, the myometrial invasion, the steroid receptor status and the lymph node status are decisive prognostic factors [15,16,17,18,19]. It has been shown that the serous papillary adenocarcinomas [20,21], adeno-squamous, clear cell, undifferentiated, steroid receptor negative carcinomas with positive lymph nodes are of an aggressive nature and are associated with a high death rate. Other parameters such as the DNA ploidy, portion of cells in S-phase, and the analysis of proto-oncogene activation can also be utilized to characterize an aggressive phenotype [22,23,24,25].

In this report we analyzed biochemically the EGF-R in different endometrial carcinomas and investigated the relationship between the EGF-R status and various clinical and histological features which have been shown to be of prognostic importance. Furthermore, the correlation between survival rates and EGF-R status was investigated in these cases.

Material and Methods

J-125-labeled EGF was purchased from Amershan-Buchler (Braunschweig, FRG) and cellulose acetate filters from Millipore (Millipore Corp., FRG). All other chemicals and reagents were of analytical grade.

Tumor Tissue

Tumor specimens were frozen in liquid nitrogen immediatly after removal and kept at -90° C until use. All tissues were examined histologically and in most specimens the estrogen (ER) and progesterone (PrR) receptors were estimated using the dextran coated charcoal method [19].

The tissue was pulverized using a dismembrator followed by a further homogenisation step in cold Tris-HCL buffer (50 mM Tris, pH 7,4, 1 mM MgCl2) with a Dounce potter. Crude plasma membranes were prepared as described [26].

The protein content of the membrane suspension was measered using the protein assay from Collaborative Research (USA) EGF-R binding assay.

EGF-R was measured by a competitive single point assay as described previously [8,9]. Briefly, the membranes were incubated in Tris-HCL buffer /0,1% bovine serum albumin pH 7,4 with 1 ng 125-I-EGF alone or together with 500 ng of unlabeled EGF. After incubation at 37° C for 45 min, unbound EGF was removed by filtration (Millipore apparatus) and the amount of specific EGF binding was calculated and corrected per mg membrane protein. The cut-off for specific EGF binding was 1 fmol/mg. Tumors with a high number of EGF binding sites expressed >10 fmol/mg.

Management of Disease and Statistics

The clinical material comprised 92 endometrial carcinomas. 80 patients were treated by surgery (73 cases with abdominal hysterectomy plus adnexe, 7 cases with vaginal hysterectomy). In 12 cases the material was received by biopsy or abrasio, and in 22 cases the pelvic lymph nodes were removed. Ten patients received a primary irradiation combination therapy with about 60 Gy cesium in contact and 50 Gy external telecobalt. Patients treated by surgery received postoperatively a vaginal iridium contact irradiation (40 Gy) and in dependence of tumor differentiation (G2,G3), myometrial invasion (>2/3) or lymph node involvement respectively, an external telecobalt irradiation (50 Gy).

The patients were followed every 3 months in the first year after the treatment and later every 6 months.

The tumor stage, histological type, grading, myometrial and parametrial invasion, lymph node status and steroid hormone receptor status were compared with the EGF-R status and statistically analyzed by a X-test. Furthermore, the survival of each patient was controlled and life table analysis was performed with log-rank test.

Results

In earlier studies we have analyzed the EGF binding parameters on different gynecologic carcinomas using the Scatchard plot and in the majority of cases found similar binding affinities between $0.5-5 \times 10^{-9}$ M but a different number of binding sites (Bmax) [8]. Therefore we decided to screen our tumor material by the easy to handle single point assay with a cut off of 1 fmol/mg. Tumors with a high number of EGF-R's had >10 fmol/mg.

EGF binding studies were performed on 92 different endometrial carcinomas with 81 primary, 3 metastatic and 8 recurrent disease cases. 48% of all tested biopsies were EGF-R(+) and 10% expressed high binding capacities (table 1). It seems that the metastasis or recurrent tumors are less frequent EGF-R(+), however, only a limited case number could be analyzed.

Table 1: Prognostic Factors and EGF Receptor Endometrial Carcinoma

Parameter:	EGF-R Status				
	EGF-R(+) All Cases	EGF-R (+) 1-10fmol	EGF-R(+) >10fmol	EGF-R(-)	Total
	Number	of	Cases	(%)	
Tumor Type:					
Primary	40 (50)	32 (40)	8 (10)	41 (50)	81 (100)
Metastatic	1 (-)	1 (-)	0 (-)	2 (-)	3 (-)
Recurrent	3 (-)	2 (-)	1 (-)	5 (-)	8 (-)
Tumor Stage:					
Stage I+II	26 (39)	22 (33)	4 (6)	41 (61)	67 (100)
Stage III+IV	18 (72)	13 (52)	5 (20)	7 (28)	25 (100)
Histology:					
Adeno	27 (47)	21 (37)	6 (10)	31 (53)	58 (100)
Adeno-acanthom	5 (60)	5 (60)	0 (-)	3 (40)	8 (100)
Adeno-squamous	3 (75)	3 (75)	0 (-)	1 (25)	4 (100)
Serous	2 (40)	2 (40)	0 (-)	3 (60)	5 (100)
Adeno-mucineous	0 (-)	0 (-)	0 (-)	1 (-)	1 (-)
Clear cell	2 (50)	2 (50)	0 (-)	2 (50)	4 (100)
Other	5 (45)	2 (18)	3 (27)	6 (55)	11 (100)
Differentiation:					
G1	12 (57)	8 (38)	4 (19)	9 (43)	21 (100)
G2	17 (59)	16 (47)	1 (3)	17 (50)	34 (100)
G3	15 (41)	11 (30)	5 (14)	22 (59)	37 (100)
Myometrial Invasion:					
< 2/3 Invas.	21 (46)	16 (35)	5 (11)	25 (54)	46 (100)
> 2/3 Invas.	17 (50)	15 (44)	2 (6)	17 (50)	34 (100)
Steroid Receptor:					
ER(+)	27 (45)	23 (38)	4 (7)	33 (55)	60 (100)
ER(-)	14 (54)	10 (39)	4 (15)	12 (46)	26 (100)
PrR(+)	28 (44)	26 (41)	2 (3)	35 (56)	63 (100)
PrR(-)	13 (57)	7 (30)	6 (27)	10 (43)	23 (100)
Lymph Node:					
LN(+)	5 (63)	4 (50)	1 (13)	3 (38)	8 (100)
LN(-)	6 (43)	6 (43)	0 (-)	8 (57)	14 (100)
Total	44 (48)	35 (38)	9 (10)	48 (52)	92 (100)

No significant difference of EGF-R frequency could be detected in correlation to the grade of differentiation or the depth of myometrial invasion respectively, as shown in table 1. Regarding the tumor stages, advanced endometrial carcinomas stage III and IV were in 60-80% EGF-R(+) compared to 30-40% in stage I and II. Furthermore, a similar tendency existed also in the findings of tumors with high binding capacities (table 1).

The distribution of histological subtypes with respect to EGF-R status are demonstrated in table 1. Endometrial cancers with a squamous cell portion, the adeno-squamous carcinomas and the adenoacanthomas, were the most frequent EGF-R(+) tumors. No difference in EGF-R expression was noticed between the adenocarcinomas and the adeno-papillary carcinomas.

Finally, the results of EGF-R and steroid hormone receptor status are shown which demonstrates an inverse correlation. ER(-) carcinomas were in 55% and PrR(-) in 58% EGF-R(+). A still more pronounced difference shows the comparison of tumors with high EGF-R binding capacities in the PrR group with 25% cases in PrR(-) tumors compared to no case in the PrR(+) group.

The survival curves of patients with endometrial carcinomas, regarding the EGF-R status alone or in combination with the tumor stage and receptor status are shown in figs. 1-3. Figure 1 shows the life table analysis of all treated patients (n=90) with respect to EGF-R status. The comparison of both curves demonstrates a small difference after an observation time over 20 months. Tumor stage, myometrial invasion and steroid receptor status are known as clinical prognostic factors. Life table analyses of EGF-R(+) and EGF-R(-) patients with respect to the specified parameters were carried out, especially those which showed a correlation with the EGF-R status (Fig. 2,3). At stage I and II again the EGF-R(+) group had a reduced survival probability, whereas no difference existed in advanced tumor stages (Fig. 2). When the groups were subdivided according to the myometrial invasion the curves were similar in the group with >2/3 myometrial invasion. In the group with no or only limited invasion (<2/3) patients with EGF-R(+) tumors seem to have a reduced survival rate (data not shown). Fig. 3 shows the life table analysis regarding ER(+) or PrR(+) tumors and the EGF-R status. No differences were found for the ER(-) or PrR(-) groups. The curves demonstrate that in the ER(+) and to a higher extend in the PrR(+) group patients with EGF-R(+) carcinomas have a poorer prognosis compared to EGF-R(-) tumor group. The data with respect to the other prognostic parameters are not shown because of the small case number.

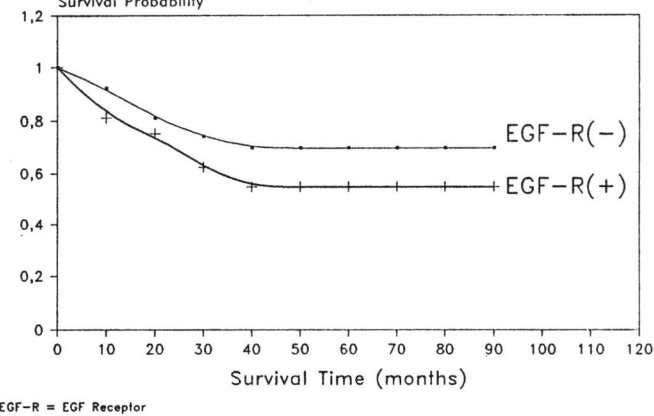

EGF-R = EGF Receptor

Figure 1: EGF-R Status and Survival Endometrial Cancer

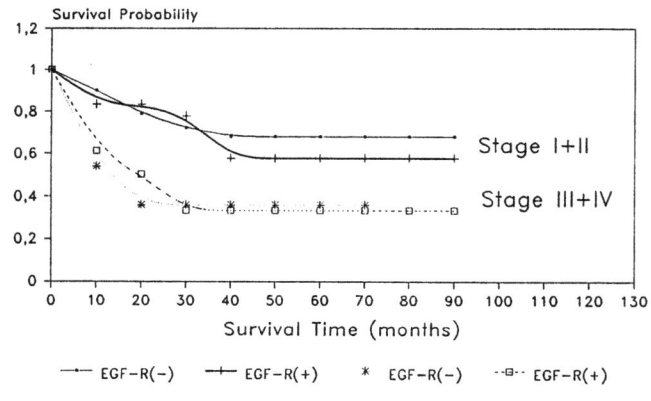

EGF-R = EGF Receptor

Figure 2: Tumor Stage and EGF Receptor Survival Curves

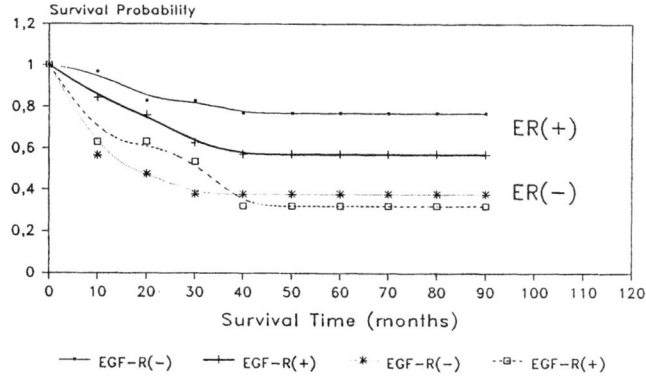

Figure 3a: Estrogen and EGF Receptor Survivial Curves

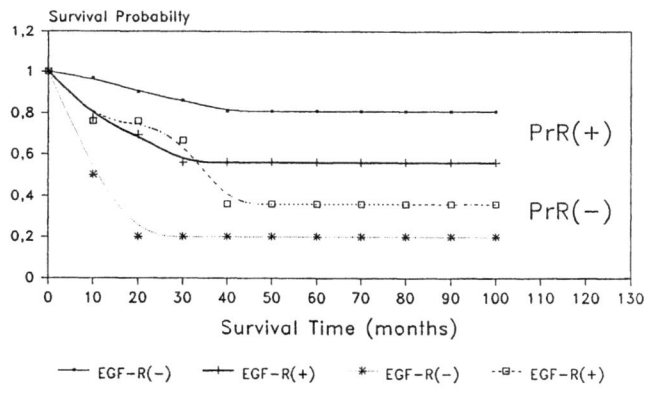

Figure 3b: Progesterone and EGF Receptors Survivial Curves

Discussion

In earlier study, we have investigated the immunohistological localization of EGF-R in different gynecologic carcinomas [26]. That study has shown that in endometrial carcinomas as well as in the other tumor types the specific EGF-R immunostaining is exclusively found in the tumor cells, whereas the stromal cells stain EGF-R(-). By the use of molecular-biochemical methods it can be seen that the amount of EGF-R expression is usually the result of a different EGF-R gene expression and not a gene modification particularly gene amplification [22]. It exists a strong correlation between the amounts of EGF-R mRNA, the staining score and the biochemical binding data [22].

This study shows that by the use of the single point EGF-R assay EGF-R(+) and EGF-R(-) endometrial carcinomas can be discriminated. 50% of these tumors are EGF-R(+) and 10% express a high number of binding sites. When we correlated the EGF-R status with established clinical prognostic factors we noticed an increased frequency of EGF-R(+) carcinomas in the advanced tumor stages and an inverse relationship to the steroid receptor status. A similar inverse correlation was also described by others for the breast carcinomas [19] and by us for the ovarian carcinomas [20]. Regarding the different histological subtypes tumors with a sqamous portion are nearly all EGF-R(+) as an expected result because squamous cell carcinomas of the cervix [27], the skin [28], the lung [29] etc. are nearly total EGF-R(+). The adenopapillary and adeno-carcinomas had similar frequencies whereas the clear cell carcinomas express a decreased EGF-R rate comparable to the ovarian carcinomas [20]. The adeno-papillary tumor types are known to correlate with poor prognosis [7]. Sasano et al. [14] found a c-myc amplification and aneuploidy in the serous papillary adenocarcinomas being consistent with its aggressive behaviour. From this it can be concluded that the EGF-R status does not discriminate these lesions with poor prognosis from the other and the investigation of oncogenes or the grade of ploidy are more relevant for these tumor types.

A further important clinical prognostic factor is the lymph node status [3]. Our investigated case number is too small for a definite conclusion but the lymph node positive tumors seem to more frequent EGF-R(+).

In the breast carcinoma the EGF-R status is an important prognostic factor for early recurrence and death especially in the ER(-) group [19]. In EGF-R(+) ovarian carcinomas we detected a significant higher response rate to chemotherapy [20,21,22]. However, the EGF-R(+) ovarian carcinomas seem to recurre early [22]. It is believed therefore that the EGF-R status signifies different aggressive phenotypes. When we performed the life table analysis of patients with endometrial carcinomas with respect to the EGF-R status and the clinical prognostic factors a reduced survival probability was noticed for the EGF-R(+) group in those collectives with a good prognosis as early tumor stages, no or minimal myometrial invasion and steroid receptor positive tumors. For the groups with poor prognosis no differences according to the EGF-R status were noticed. In comparison to the breast at which groups with poor prognosis can further be subdivided by the EGF-R status, a similar discrimination can be performed for the endometrial carcinomas however only for the groups with good prognostic parameters. The problem in the treatment of endometrial carcinomas with good prognosis is probably an overtreatment in some cases. For the future we hope with a higher case number to define these groups better allowing a safe conservative treatment procedure.

References

1. Garrett C (1986) Oncogenes. Clin Chim Acta 156: 1-40
2. Merkel DE, McGuire WL (1988) Oncogenes and cancer prognosis. In: Devita VT Jr, Hellmann S, Rosenberg eds: Important advances in oncology. Philadelphia: Lippincott JB, pp 103-117
3. Downward J, Yarden Y, Mayes E, Scrace G, Totty N et al (1984) Close similarity of epidermal growth factor receptor and v-erb B oncogene protein sequences.Nature 307: 521-527
4. Carpenter G and Cohen S (1979) Epidermal growth factor. Ann Rev Biochem 48: 193-216
5. Massaque J (1983) Epidermal growth factor like transforming growth factor. J Biol Chem 258: 13606-13614
6. Derynck R (1986) Transforming growth factor structure and biological activities. J Cell Biochem 32: 293-304
7. Sainsbury J, Farndorn J, Needham G, Malcolm A, and Harris A (1987) Epidermal growth factor receptor status as predictor for early recurrence of and death from breast cancer. Lancet I: 1398-1402
8. Bauknecht T, Runge M, Schwall M, and Pfleiderer A (1988) Occurrence of epidermal growth factor receptor in human adnexal tumors and their prognostic value in advanced ovarian carcinomas. Gynecol Oncol 29:147-159

9. Bauknecht T, Janz I, Kohler M, and Pfleiderer A (1989) Human ovarian carcinomas: Correlation of malignancy and survival with the expression of epidermal growth factor receptor and EGF like factor. Med Oncol Pharmacother 6: 121-127
10. Kohler M, Janz I, Wintzer HO, Wagner E, Bauknecht T (1989) The expression of epidermal growth factor receptor, EGF like factors and c-myc in ovarian and cervical carcinomas and their potential clinical significance. Anticancer Res 9: 1537-1548
11. Hunts I, Ueda M, Ozawa S, Abe O, Pastan I and Shimizu N (1985) Hyperproduction and gene amplification of the epidermal growth factor receptor in squamous cell carcinomas. Jpn. J. Cancer Res 76: 663-666
12. Yasui M, Sumgoski H, Hata I, Kameda I, Ochiai A, Ito H, and Tahara E (1988) Expression of epidermal growth factor receptor in human gastric and colonic carcinoma. Cancer Res 48: 137-141
13. Keski-Oja J, Leof E, Lyons R, Coffey R, Moses H (1987) Transforming growth factors and control of neoplastic cell growth. J Cell Biochem 33: 95-107
14. Kistner RW (1979) Adenocarcinoma. In: Gynecologic Principles and Practise, Chicago: Year Book Medical Publisher, Inc., pp 255-272
15. Aalders JG, Abeler V, and Kolstad P (1984) Clinical (stage III) as compared to subclinical intrapelvic extrauterine tumor spread in endometrial carcinoma: A clinical and histopathological study of 175 patients. Gynecol Oncol 17: 64-74
16. Chambers SK, Kapp DS, Peschel RE, Lawrence R, Mernio M, Kohoru EI, Schwarz PE (1987) Prognostic factors and sites of failure in Figo stage I, grade 3 endometrial cancer. Gynocol Oncol 27: 180-188
17. Grisgby PW, Perez CA, Kushe RR, Kao MS, and Galakatos AE (1987) Results of therapy, analysis of failures and prognostic factors for clinical and pathological stage III adenocarcinoma of the endometrium. Gynocol Oncol 27: 44-57
18. Goff BA, and Rice LW (1990) Assessment of depth of myometrial invasion in endometrial adenocarcinoma. Gynecol Oncol 38: 46-48
19. Kleine W, Maier T, Geyer H, and Pfleiderer A (1990) Estrogen and progesterone receptors in endometrial cancer and their prognostic relevance. Gynecol Oncol 38: 59-65
20. Hendrickson M, Ross J, Eifel P, Martinez A, Kempson R (1982) Uterine papillary serous carcinoma: A highly malignant form of endometrial carcinoma. Am J Surg Pathol 6: 93-108
21. Sutton GP, Brill L, Michael H, Stehmann FB, Ehrlich CE (1987) Malignant papillary lesions of the endometrium. Gynecol Oncol 27: 294-304

22. Sorbe B, Risberg B, and Frankendal B (1990) DNA ploidy, morphometry and nuclear grade as prognostic factors in endometrial carcinoma. Gynecol Oncol 38: 22-27
23. Friedlander M, Hedley DW, Taylor I (1984) Clinical and biological significance of aneuploidy in human tumors. J. Clin. Pathol. 37: 961-974
24. Tsou KC, Hong DH, Varello MA et al. (1985) Flow cytometric DNA and 5'nucleotide phosphodiesterase in endometrium. Cancer 56: 2340-2347
25. Sasano H, Comeford J, Wilkinson D, Schwartz A, Garrett C (1990) Serous papillary adenocarcinoma of the endometrium: Analysis of proto-oncogene amplification, flow cytometry, estrogen and progesterone receptors, and immunohistochemistry. Cancer 65: 1545-1551
26. Bauknecht T, Rau B, Meerpohl HG, Pfleiderer A (1984) The prognostic value of the presence of epidermal growth factor receptor in ovarian carcinomas. Tumor Diagnostik Therapie 5: 62-66
27. Wittmaack FM, Schwörer D, Wintzer HO, von Kleist S, Pfleiderer A, Bauknecht T (1988) The immunohistochemical investigation of epidermal growth factor receptor in various gynecological tumors. IJIPP 1: 139-147
28. Bauknecht T, Kohler M, Janz I, Pfleiderer A (1989) The occurrence of epidermal growth factor receptor and the characterisation of EGF like factors in human ovarian, endometrial, cervical and breast cancer. J Cancer Res Clin Oncol 115: 193-199
29. Bauknecht T, Gross G, Hagedorn M (1985) Epidermal growth factor receptor in different skin tumors. Dermatologica 171: 16-20
30. Veale D, Marsh C, Ashcroft T, Harris A (1985) Epidermal growth factor receptor in non-small cell lung cancer. Br J Cancer 52: 441

On Hereditary Factors in Endometrial Carcinoma

S. Kullander

A number of findings justifies the assertion that hereditary factors are crucially involved in several cases of endometrial carcinoma.

A high incidence of familial aggregation in cancer may be due either to random clustering of sporadic cases, shared exposure to environmental carcinogens, hereditary factors or a combination of any of these. It is still common to view cancer cases as random or »sporadic« phenomena. Such comments as »No familial aspects of any relevance« used to be standard blocks in our medical records. A tumour that might at first glance appear to be a »sporadic« case may nonetheless have strong hereditary connotations.

In various hereditary cancer syndromes particularly those with breast cancer, ovarian cancer, or non-polyposis (usually rightsided) colon cancer – the characteristic features have been early tumour onset and high incidence of multiple primary tumours among family members. A very heterogenous multiple tumour spectrum, with varying expression of the defective gene, sometimes even including malformation, is now considered to be characteristic of cancer families, and to be due to a hereditary cancerpredisposing factor.

Variation in the numbers of relatives and variation in family size and in the interrelations with environmental factors may explain differences in individual and pedigree cancer frequency and distribution, even in cases of the same genetic defect.

Population studies are essential, if misleading bias is to be avoided when determining the significance of familial or genetic factors. Endometrial cancer has been shown to be associated with a variety of constitutional entities such as diabetes, obesity, and hypertension.

However, no systematic studies have been made of the occurrence of the same endometrial cancer form, or of other cancer forms, in kindreds. Thus, the approach that seemed to be indicated was that of a controlled epidemiological case-control study of endometrial cancer to be succeeded by chromosomal and molecular studies. Malmö is particularly well suited to such studies. Its population of 240.000 is large enough yet manageable, and it is served by a single hospital to which all tumour cases are remitted and where they are subsequently followed up. The population ist fairly static and easily accessible for the purposes of information, collection or distribution, and the autopsy frequency is high.

To avoid confusion due to small histological subgroups, detailed analysis was confined to cases of adenocarcinoma – by far the predominant type of malignancy in endometrial cancer. The series comprised all newly diagnosed cases of endometrial adenocarcinoma treated at Malmö during a two-year period. While attending the clinic patients were interviewed in connection with a review answers to a standardized questionnaire on family history. The questionnaire had been distributed in advance to allow patients ample time for contacting and questioning members of their families. Information was collected of malignant disease and malformation for all first degree relatives, both of the patients and their consorts, which were chosen as controls. As far as possible, all reported instances of cancer were checked with the help of medical record and histopathology and autopsy reports.

At a review two years after the interview study, each case was checked with regard to histopathology, and whether the patients was symptom-free, had suffered recurrence of endometrial cancer, or had died of it. All patients had been given the routine treatment for this cancer, standard at the clinic. In the two-year series of altogether 51 patients investigated Malmö, additional primary malignancy occurred in nine cases (18%), in one of which there were two additional primary malignancies (one mammary, the other on skin cancer). The other additional primary carcinomas had occurred in the breast or cervix, and predated the endometrial cancer – and in three cases occurring simultaneously it was ovarian cancer.

In the series as a whole (n=51), cancer was present in a first degree relative in 26 cases; and of the total of 230 relatives, cancer occurred in 41, or 17,9% – which is significantly more than corresponding figure of 9,4% for the relatives of controls.

Age at onset was lower among endometrial cancer patients whose cancer predisposition was seemingly inherited from the father, than in those where it was seemingly inherited from the mother.

Not only was the incidence of cancer higher among relatives of endometrial cancer patients than among affected relatives of controls, but age at onset was lower. The difference in incidence is due to a higher rate of cancer in organs particularly sensitive to hormonal changes - the genital tract, the breast, and the prostate; but it is also due to a high incidence of cancer of the colon. Endometrial cancer occurred in four mothers or sisters of probands; and where histological findings were reviewed we found identical patterns of poorly differentiated adenocarcinoma in the proband and her sister.

In general, endometrial cancer manifesting multiple malignancy or familial cancer predisposition was associated with poorly differentiated adenocarcinoma of advanced stage and poorer prognosis.

The epidemiological findings outlined suggest the familial presence of a mutated endometrial gene in around 10% of all cases of adenocarcinoma of the uterine body. No genetic studies with modern recombinant DNA techniques seem to have been done so far in connection with endometrial cancer. Until proper DNA probes are available, such simple and readily performed measures as the taking of a thorough family history are of crucial importance. Familial aggregation of endometrial cancer or suspected genetic cancer predisposition in the patient should alert the physician to the necessity of extra care, also in the surveillance of members of the family.

It is my personal philosophy that, in such family members, the use of oestrogens for contraceptive or anti-climacteric purposes is to be avoided, as expression of an endometrial oncogene may well be hormone-dependent and oestrogen-associated.

Endometrial cancer is known as a heterogenic picture in women belonging to families exhibiting Cancer Family Syndrome, CFS. This syndrome seems more common that has hitherto been assumed. The epidemiological findings in Malmö indicate that occurrence of several »fragments« of the syndrome in the population. It is interesting that other cancers in hormone-sensitive genital tissues may be heterogenic manifestations as well. Such tumours appeared also both in the pedigrees and as double primaries in the endometrial cancer cases studied. Regarding our findings, it should be noticed that Peutz-Jegher's syndrome, a rare hereditary disorder with gastrointestinal polyposis associated with characteristic skin pigmentation, has an increased risk for the development of cancer of the colon but also of ovarian cancer, sometimes with a rather specific histologic picture with anular tubules, causing hyperestrinisme [1,2]. A distincitive stromal ovarian tumour also has been described in connection with Peutz-Jegher [3] as well as mucinous adenocarcinomas of the cervix uteri [1]. Accordingly in health surveillance of women belonging to families manifesting more or less obvious CSF extra attention should be given to genital organs.

References

1. Young RH, Welch WR, Dickersin GR and Scully RE: Cancer 50 :1384, 1982
2. Utsunomiya J, Gocho H, Miyanaga T, Hamaguchi E, Kashimure A, Aoki N and Komatsu I. The Johns Hopkins Med J 136: 71, 1975
3. Young RH, Dickersin GR and Scully RE, Am J Surg Pathol 7: 233, 1983

III. Operatives Vorgehen

Surgery for Endometrial Carcinoma

Neville F. Hacker

The past decade has witnessed significant advances in our knowledge of endometrial cancer. Careful surgical staging has more clearly elucidated spread patterns of early disease, and prognostic variables have been better defined. This has allowed more individualization of treatment.

The cornerstone of treatment remains total abdominal hysterectomy and bilateral salpingo-oophorectomy, and this operation should be performed for all cases whenever feasible. Several studies have demonstrated that patients treated with radiation alone have a significantly inferior survival to patients treated surgically [1,2,3], unlike the situation with cervical cancer, where surgery and radiation are equally efficacious.

It is desirable to remove the ovaries as well as the uterus, because they may be a site of microscopic metastases, they may produce »unopposed« estrogen in premenopausal patients, and patients with endometrial cancer are at increased risk for primary ovarian cancer. Such tumors sometimes occur concurrently [4].

It has been common practice to use preoperative radiation for patients with endometrial cancer. One of the proposed advantages has been that the radiation will sterilize the malignant cells, thereby decreasing the likelihood of vaginal implantation or systemic dissemination at the time of hysterectomy. However, Truskett and Constable reported a vaginal recurrence rate of 6,2% for patients with no residual disease in the operative specimen following preoperative intrauterine Heyman Capsules, strongly suggesting that vaginal metastases result from lymphatic spread, rather than implantation [5]. In addition, Bean et al reported distant metastases in four of 130 (3%) patients treated with preoperative radiation, compared with one of 150 (0,7%) patients treated with primary surgery [6]. These data suggest that primary surgery is not a significant risk factor for systemic dissemination.

Table 1: Absolute Indications for Primary Surgery

1. Pelvic or abdominal mass
2. Ascites
3. Prior pelvic abscess
4. Pyometra
5. Stage I, Grade I tumors
6. Unreliable patient

Postoperative radiation allows the type of radiation to be individualized according to the operative findings. It also means that radiation can be eliminated in well differentiated tumors with less than one-third of myometrial invasion. Some workers, including those at the Radiumhemmet, continue to advocate preoperative brachytherapy for patients with grade 3 histology [7]. Absolute indications for primary surgery are shown in Table 1.

Operative Technique

The following technique is appropriate for all patients with Stage I and occult Stage II disease (ie: cervix not grossly involved).

The laparotomy is best performed through a lower midline incision, particularly for patients with unfavourable histologies (Table 2). The incidence of extrauterine spread in patients with an unfavourable histology was reported by Wilson and colleagues from the Mayo Clinic, to be 62% [8], so full surgical staging is required. Omentectomy, removal of enlarged paraaortic nodes, or resection of abdominal metastases may also be required in patients with an enlarged uterus, cervical extension, or an adnexal mass [9], so a midline incision is also desirable for these patients. In the presence of obesity and a large abdominal panniculus, which is not uncommon in patients with endometrial carcinoma, a lower midline incision may offer better exposure [10].

On entering the abdomen, peritoneal washings are taken for cytology from the pelvis, paracolic gutters, and subdiaphragmatic area, using 50 ml of normal saline. Thorough exploration of the abdomen is then performed, noting particularly the liver, diaphragm, omentum and paraaortic nodes.

Table 2: The Unfavourable Histologies

1. Poorly or undifferentiated tumors
2. Adenosquamous
3. Papillary Serous
4. Clear Cell
5. Squamous

Table 3: Patients Requiring Surgical Staging

1. Unfavourable histologic type
2. > 50% myometrial invasion
3. Cervical extension

Extrafascial hysterectomy is performed after dividing the round ligaments and carrying the peritoneal incision anteriorly around the vesicouterine fold and posteriorly parallel and lateral to the infundibulopelvic ligaments. With a narrow Deaver retractor in the retroperitoneum providing gentle traction cephaled in the direction of the common iliac vessels, each ureter is displayed and the infundibulopelvic ligaments are divided and ligated. The bladder is dissected off the front of the cervix then the uterine vessels are skeletonized and divided at the level of the isthmus. Straight Kocher forceps are used to secure the cardinal and uterosacral ligaments, and angled clamps are used to secure the vaginal vault. No cuff of vagina is taken. The uterus, tubes, and ovaries are removed and the vault closed.

The specimen is opened on the operating table, and possible cervical extension and myometrial invasion are evaluated. Surgical staging is indicated for patients shown on Table 3.

Surgical Staging

The new FIGO staging for endometrial cancer is based on surgical staging.

Thorough surgical staging requires peritoneal washings for cytology, biopsy of any suspicious extrauterine nodules, infracolic omentectomy, multiple peritoneal biopsies as is done for ovarian cancer, together with bilateral pelvic lymphadenectomy.

Although surgical staging is the ideal way to divide patients into prognostic groups, there are several difficulties with making this a universal requirement in patients with endometrial cancer:

1. The majority of patients with endometrial cancer are not treated by gynaecological oncologists, so the treating physician will not be trained in the techniques of lymphadenectomy.

Lymphadenectomy in the hands of an untrained surgeon is likely to be both morbid and inadequate. However, it is difficult to justify a recommendation that all patients with endometrial cancer should be referred to cancer centres for primary surgery, because patients with a normal sized uterus, no cervical extension, no adnexal mass, and favourable (well differentiated) histology will have an excellent prognosis in the hands of a general gynaecologist, with postoperative adjuvant pelvic radiation offered on the basis of histologic differentiation and depth of myometrial penetration.

2. Many patients with endometrial cancer are obese and medically unfit and not suitable candidates for extensive lymphadenectomies, even in the hands of trained oncologists.

3. To be reliable, a lymphadenectomy must be complete. Sampling of selected nodes will inevitably result in false negative nodal evaluations.

As a consequence of the above factors, most patients with endometrial cancer will be inadequately staged by the new FIGO criteria.

Although surgical staging protocols such as those of the Gynecologic Oncology Group in the United States have provided important information on prognostic factors and patterns of spread, it has not been demonstrated that full lymphadenectomy offers any therapeutic advantage over resection of enlarged lymph nodes and adjuvant radiation.

In addition, as the hysterectomy is an extrafascial procedure without resection of parametrium, elimination of pelvic radiation in a patient with high risk factors in the uterus but negative pelvic nodes may increase the risk of central recurrence. For the above reasons, the author's current approach to the lymph nodes in patients with endometrial cancer is as follows:

1. All pelvic and paraaortic nodes are carefully palpated, and any enlarged nodes are resected. Full dissection is not performed.

2. If no positive nodes are identified the decision regarding the need for adjuvant pelvic radiation is based on the histologic type, differentiation, and depth of myometrial invasion.

3. If pelvic nodal metastases are identified, pelvic and paraaortic radiation is given, as approximately two-thirds of patients with positive pelvic nodes will have positive paraaortic nodes [11].

Stage II Endometrial Cancer

Two main approaches have been used for patients with Stage II endometrial cancer:

1. Radical hysterectomy, bilateral salpingo-oophorectomy, and bilateral pelvic lymphadenectomy.

2. Preoperative external pelvic radiation, one intracavitary cesium, followed by total abdominal hysterectomy and bilateral salpingo-oopherectomy 6 weeks later.

Both protocols fail to address the problem of extrapelvic spread. The incidence of metastases to paraaortic lymph nodes, adnexal structures and upper abdomen would be expected to be higher for Stage II lesions, but surgical staging data are not available.

The author's approach to patients with gross cervical involvement is as follows [12]:

1. Modified radical hysterectomy and bilateral salpingo-oophorectomy.
2. Pelvic and abdominal peritoneal washings.

3. Infracolic omentectomy.
4. Resection of any suspicious extrauterine nodules.
5. Resection of grossly enlarged pelvic or paraaortic lymph nodes.
6. If there are no enlarged nodes, resection of common iliac and lower paraaortic nodes.

All patients receive postoperative pelvic radiation, and paraaortic radiation is added if any positive pelvic or paraaortic nodes are identified.

Special Situations

1. Stage III disease: Treatment for Stage III endometrial cancer must be individualized, but should include total abdominal hysterectomy and bilateral salpingo-oophorectomy. In the presence of an adnexal mass, surgery should be performed initially to determine the nature of the mass and to remove the bulk of the disease. In the presence of parametrial extension, it will usually be more appropriate to commence with external radiation and intracavitary cesium. Surgical eradication of all macroscopic tumor is of major prognostic importance in patients with Stage III disease [13].

2. Stage IV disease: Treatment for Stage IV disease must be individualized, but will usually involve a combination of surgery, radiation therapy and progestins. The objective of surgery is to try to achieve local disease control in the pelvis, in order to help palliate bleeding, discharge, and complications involving the bowel and bladder. Aalders [14] reported that control of the pelvic disease could be achieved in 20 of 72 patients (28%) using radiation alone or in combination with surgery and/or progestins.

3. Synchronous primary tumors in the endometrium and ovary: In about half such cases, both endometrial and ovarian tumors will be of the endometrioid type. The patients are often premenopausal, and have a favourable prognosis. Treatment should be determined on the basis that each represents a primary lesion, and many will require surgery only, without adjuvant radiation [4]. Careful surgical staging, as for ovarian cancer, is important in such cases. If the histologies are more aggressive or dissimilar, the prognosis is worse, and adjuvant radiation should be used.

4. Well differentiated carcinomas in very young women: Such lesions usually occur in association with the Stein Levanthal Syndrome, and in 90% of cases are well differentiated histologically, with limited, if any,

myometrial invasion [15]. A two-month trial of high-dose progestins may be undertaken if childbearing is desired, and if repeat curettage in 2 months shows no evidence of carcinoma, conservative treatment may continue. If the lesion persists, or if childbearing is not desired, hysterectomy is the treatment of choice [16,17]. Castration in these young patients may be avoided [16]. Lesions other than well differentiated adenocarcinomas should be treated in the standard manner.

5. Vaginal Hysterectomy: In selected patients with marked obesity and medical problems that place them at high risk for abdominal operations, vaginal hysterectomy is preferable to radiation therapy. It is particularly applicable to patients with Grade I lesions [18,19].

Conclusions

Endometrial cancer should be treated with surgery primarily, whenever feasible. In addition to total abdominal hysterectomy and bilateral salpingo-oophorectomy, surgical staging in high risk patients and resection of all gross disease should be the goals of surgical management. Complete pelvic lymphadenectomy, with or without paraaortic lymphadenectomy, is not feasible for many patients, and has no proven therapeutic value. Surgical staging protocols involving lymph node dissections have identified patterns of spread and risk factors for nodal involvement, and adjuvant radiation can now be given on the basis of known prognostic variables.

References

1. Bickenbach W, Lochmuller H, Dirlich G et al: Factor analysis of endometrial carcinoma in relation to treatment. Obstet Gynecol 29: 632, 1967
2. Joelsson I, Sandri A, Kottmeier HL: Carcinoma of the uterine corpus: a retrospective survey of individualized therapy. Acta Radiol (Suppl) 334: 3, 1973
3. Grigsby PW, Perez CA, Camel HM, Galakatos AE: Stage II carcinoma of the endometruim: results of therapy and prognostic factors. Int J Radiat Oncol Biol Phys 11: 1915, 1985
4. Eiffel P, Hendrickson M, Ross J et al: Simultaneous presentation of carcinoma involving the ovary and the uterine corpus. Cancer 50: 163, 1982

5. Truskett ID, Constable WC: Management of carcinoma of the corpus uteri. Am J Obstet Gynecol 101: 689, 1968
6. Bean HA, Bryant AS, Carmichael JA, Mallik A: Carcinoma of the endometrium in Saskatchewan: 1966 to 1971. Gynecol Oncol 6: 503, 1978
7. Surwit EA, Joelsson I, Einhorn N: Adjuvant radiation therapy in the management of stage I cancer of the endometrium. Obstet Gynecol 58: 590, 1981
8. Wilson TO, Podratz KC, Gaffey TA et al:Evaluation of unfavourable histologic subtypes in endometrial adenocarcinoma. Am J Obstet Gynecol 162: 418, 1990
9. Morrow CP, Schlaerth JB: Surgical management of endometrial carcinoma. Clin Obstet Gynecol 25: 81, 1982
10. Morrow CP, Hernandez WL, Townsend DE, DiSaia PJ: Pelvic celiotomy in the obese patient. Am J Obstet Gynecol 127: 335, 1977
11. Boronow RC, Morrow CP, Creasman WT et al: Surgical staging in endometrial cancer: Clinicopathologic findings of a prospective study. Obstet Gynecol 63: 825, 1984
12. Hacker NF: Endometrial Cancer. In Practical Gynecologic Oncology: Berek JS, Hacker NF (Eds) Williams and Wilkins, Baltimore, 1989
13. Aalders J, Abeler V, Kolstad P: Clinical (Stage III) as compared to subclinical intrapelvic extrauterine tumor spread in endometrial carcinoma: a clinical and histopathological study of 175 patients. Gynecol Oncol 17: 64, 1984
14. Aalders J, Abeler V, Kolstad P:Stage IV endometrial carcinoma: a clinical and histopathological study of 83 patients. Gynecol Oncol 17: 75, 1984
15. Farhi DC, Nosanchuk J, Silberberg SG: Endometrial adenocarcinoma in women under 25 years of age. Obstet Gynecol 68: 741, 1986
16. Kempson RL, Pokorny GE: Adenocarcimoma of the endometrium in women aged forty and younger. Cancer 21: 650, 1968
17. Fechner RE, Kaufman RH: Endometrial adenocarcimoma in Stein-Levanthal Syndrome. Cancer 34: 444, 1974
18. Peters WA III, Andersen WA, Thornton N Jr, Morley GW: The selective use of vaginal hysterectomy in the management of adenocarcinoma of the endometrium. Am J Obstet Gynecol 146: 285, 1983
19. Malkasian GD, Annegers JF, Pountain KS: Carcinoma of the endometrium: stage I. Am J Obstet Gynecol 136: 872, 1980

Treatment of Clinical Early Endometrial Carcinoma; Indications for Lymphonodectomy

J. Aalders

Introduction

A multitude of treatment regimes for endometrial carcinoma has been reported in the last decades. Surgery, consisting of a total hysterectomy and bilateral salpingo-oophorectomy is generally accepted as the cornerstone in the management of early endometrial carcinoma. When radiotherapy proved to be also effective in the management of endometrial cancer, the combined therapy, using both irradiation and surgery, became the most commonly performed treatment for endometrial cancer. However, the type and timing of additional radiotherapy, especially in the early stages of endometrial cancer, still remains controversial. This is clearly illustrated in the 1988 Annual Report on the results of treatment in gynecologic cancer (Table 1).

The general feeling that combined therapy, using both surgery and radiotherapy, is superior to surgery alone has never been documented. In his thorough review including 6071 cases from 23 reports, Jones [2] found no difference between the five-year survival for patients with stage I disease treated by surgery (75%) or combined therapy (78%). However the results may be biased by the lack of adequate information of histologic grade and depth of myometrial invasion. It is obvious that patients with poorly differentiated and deeply infiltrating tumors are likely to be overpresented numbers in the combined treatment group.

The only prospective study to evaluate the value of postoperative pelvic radiotherapy as standard therapy for all patients with FIGO stage I endometrial cancer has been performed at the Norwegian Radium Hospital and reported by Aalders et al. (1980) [3]. After primary surgery all 540 patients received vaginal radium delivering 6000 rads to the vaginal vault. The patients were then randomized in controls, receiving no further treatment and those receiving additional high voltage external radiotherapy to a pelvic field with a dose of 4000 rads to the pelvic lymph nodes.

Table 1: Reported treatment modalities for stage I

	Patients	
Surgery alone	1.692	(15,3%)
Surgery + post operative radiation	4.233	(38,4%)
Preoperative radiation	4.518	(40,9%)
Radiation alone or hormonal and/or chemotherapy	592	(5,4%)
Total	11.035	(100%)

Adapted from Pettersson, F. (ed.): Annual Report on the results of treatment in gynecologic cancer, vol. 20, Stockholm (1988) FIGO [1]

During the follow-up period of 3 to 10 years a significant reduction in vaginal and pelvic recurrences was found in the patients receiving additional pelvic radiation as compared with the controls (1,9 versus 6,9%, p<0,01). However this was outweighed by the higher number of distant metastases in women who received pelvic radiation (9,9%) compared to the controls (5,4%) leading to comparable 5-year survival rates (91% for controls and 89% for patients receiving additional pelvic radiation).

A more detailed analysis of this series led to the conclusion that only patients with poorly differentiated tumors (grade 3), which infiltrate more than half the myometrial thickness, might benefit from additional external radiotherapy. The disappointing results of the combination with additional postoperative pelvic radiotherapy are obvious since we have disposal of the data of the surgical-pathologic G.O.G. study, indicating a substantial number of patients with extra pelvic disease in clinical stage I. Both local vaginal radiation and external irradiation are effective in reducing the incidence of vaginal vault recurrences. Lotocki et al. [4] reported that preoperative or postoperative vault radium decreased the incidence of vault recurrence from 14% to 1,7%. Piver et al. [5], compared hysterectomy only, preoperative uterine radium plus hysterectomy and hysterectomy plus postoperative vaginal radium in a randomized trial of 189 patients with stage I disease. They found no vaginal recurrences in the postoperative vaginal radium group, compared with a 4,5% incidence for the preoperative uterine radium patients and 7,5% for the hysterectomy only patients.

These and other data have contributed to a trend toward postoperative rather than preoperative radiation in stage I endometrial cancer. Optimal individual treatment is accomplished best when all significant surgical-pathologic information is available and both under- and overtreatment can be avoided.

Suggested treatment by stage

Stage I and stage II occult

The initial approach should be an extra facial total abdominal hysterectomy and bilateral salpingo-oophorectomy, preferably by a midline suprapubic incision. Suture closure of the cervix over an alcohol gauze, to prevent spillage of tumor cells during surgery, has been abandoned. No study has ever demonstrated that this procedure contributed to a reduction in vaginal recurrences or in an improved survival. Besides, the origin of vaginal vault recurrences from spread during surgery has been disputed. The vaginal (vault) recurrences are more likely to be the result of lymphatic spread prior to hysterectomy [6]. For the same reason a wide vaginal cuff does not seem to contribute to a reduction in vaginal recurrences.

A sample for peritoneal cytology should be obtained immediately upon entering the peritoneal cavity, either by aspiration of the fluid present or after irrigating the peritoneal cavity with saline solution.

A careful exploration of the abdominal cavity is performed, including the liver, diaphragm, omentum, pelvic and paraaortic nodes. All suspicious lesions should be biopsed.

As soon as the uterus is removed it should be opened to visualize the tumor. Frequently the extent of the tumor, in respect to myometrial invasion and expansion to isthmus or cervix is easily to assess with the naked eye. If there is a question about it, the pathologist is asked to make an assessment by frozen section.

For the aortic node sampling it is preferable to reflect the cecum and the right colon to expose retroperitoneally the lower aorta and the vena cava. This approach minimizes the likehood of small bowel adhesions in the area of the aortic node dissection and leading to intestinal complications from additional extended-field radiotherapy.

Additional surgical staging, including pelvic node dissection and selective paraaortic node sampling is performed in patients with the following unfavourable prognostic characteristics:

- patients with adenosquamous, clearcell or papillary serous carcinomas
- patients with tumor spread to cervix and/or adnexa
- patients with tumor invasion of the myometrium:
    - inner 1/3   – grade 3
    - middle 1/3   – grades 2 and 3
    - outer 1/3   – grades 1, 2 and 3
- patients with an elevated pretreatment serum CA 125 level.

Vaginal hysterectomy for endometrial carcinoma has been reported by several authors. This approach may be advantageous for certain patients at high risk (obesity, high age, poor medical condition). The vaginal procedure is often less time consuming and less traumatic as compared to an abdominal operation. However, vaginal removal of the adnexa is not always easily performed and frequently not possible at all and one is deprived of careful and thorough exploration of the abdomen, including the lymph nodes. Therefore, in view of our present knowledge, one should be reserved by performing a vaginal hysterectomy.

Additional radiotherapy

The recommended treatment plan is illustrated in figure 1.

The excellent prognosis for patients with grade 1 lesions invading less than the inner 1/3 of the myometrium does not warrant adjuvant irradiation. If, after surgical staging in the high risk patient, both the pelvic and aortic nodes prove to be free of metastatic disease, the risk is not high enough to justify irradiation of the entire pelvis, including the pelvic wall.

However, irradiation by vaginal ovoids will not result in an adequate dose to the paracervical and parametrial tissues and therefore a small-field external beam treatment would be even better to reduce the incidence of local recurrences.

Extended field irradiation should be reserved for patients with histologic proven aortic node metastases, in the absence of other extrapelvic intraperitoneal metastases.

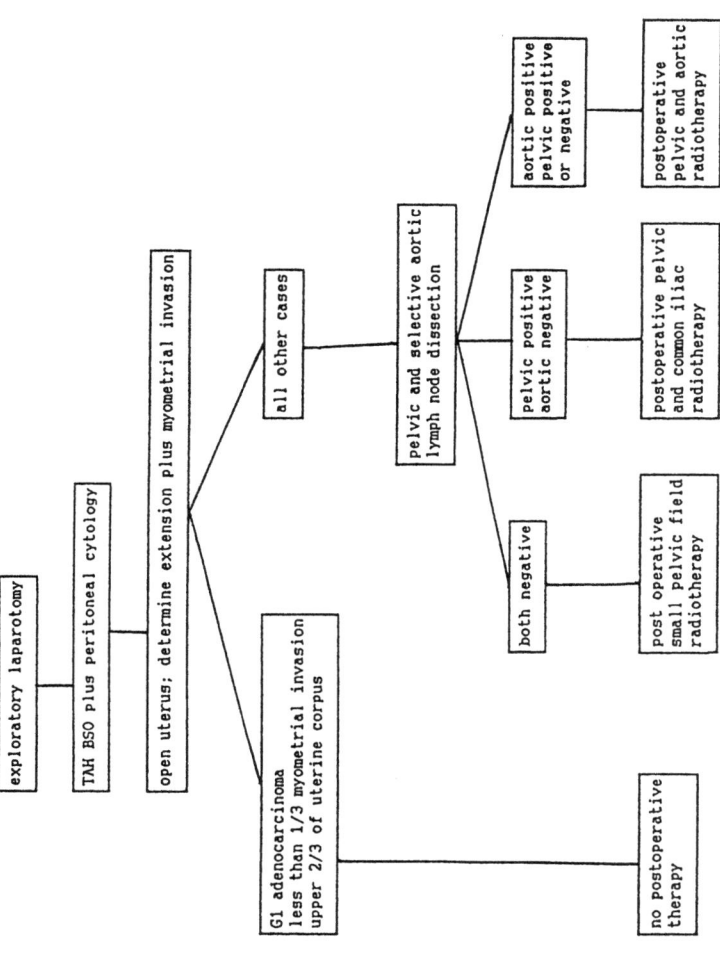

Figure 1: Management of patients with stage I and II occult endometrial carcinoma
TAH BSO: Total abdominal hysterectomy and bilateral salpingo-oophorectomy.
Source: Morrow CP, Townsend DE [16] and Aalders JG [17].

Potish et al. [7] reported 45% three year survival in aortic node positive cases in an uncontrolled series, using modern techniques of extended field irradiation. No severe morbidity has been observed in his series.

In the presence of multiple or enlarged aortic node metastases, the scalene fat pad should be removed. Metastases at that level would be a contraindication to extended field radiation therapy to the para-aortic area.

Positive peritoneal cytology

The presence of abundant malignant cells in the peritoneal cytology sample, seriously affects prognosis. This makes it imperative to design a treatment plan that might prevent recurrences. Preliminary results, as presented by Creasman et al. [8], using intraperitoneal P-32 and by Piver [9], using progesterone therapy, are encouraging. Whole-abdominal radiation therapy may be preferable for patients who have additional indications for pelvic and aortic field irradiation.

Without definite data, active treatment for patients with positive peritoneal cytology should be conducted only in a research setting.

Adjuvant progestagens

Since progesterone appeared to be effective in the treatment of recurrent or advanced endometrial adenocarcinoma, studies to test the drug in an adjuvant setting in early stage endometrial cancer became logical. However, experience from collected series has not demonstrated a significant effect of such treatment [10,11]. The major difficulty with such studies is the very high number of patients needed to detect statistically reliable differences in recurrence rate, since the overall survival is relatively good and no more than one third of these tumors are responding on progestagens.

A prospective randomized trial, to study the contribution of adjuvant medroxy progesteron acetate (400 mg Provera^R daily), in high risk stage I endometrial carcinoma patients, is presently conducted by the Clinical Oncology Society of Australia [12]. This study might give an answer to the value of adjuvant progestagens in stage I high risk patients.

Stage II

When endometrial carcinoma extends into the cervix it becomes accessable to the lower uterine vasculature and may metastasize by way of the cervical lymphatics. The incidence of pelvic node metastases is higher in stage II (35%) compared with stage I (11%) endometrial carcinoma [13]. The chances of parametrial and upper vaginal tumor extension and pelvic node metastasis make the stage II patient a more likely candidate for the radical hysterectomy and pelvic lymphadenectomy. However, modern megavoltage irradiation has proved to be effective in destroying metastatic sites of adenocarcinoma in the parametrium, upper vagina and pelvic nodes. Therefore, many gynecologists prefer to perform a conventional extrafascial hysterectomy in combination with radiotherapy in these older patients who are frequently at a poor-medical risk.

In his detailed review on this subject Rutledge [14] concluded that a more extended treatment is mandatory for most patients with stage II disease. However, no superior treatment regimen could be selected from the available literature.

From the Oslo stage II study [15] it was found to be of prognostic significance if there was microscopic or grossly visible tumor involvement of the cervix. The latter group had a higher death and recurrence rate (40%) as compared to patients with microscopic tumor involvement of the cervix (17.5%; $0.05 < P < 0.10$). The survival and recurrence rate for patients with microscopic cervical involvement was comparable with that reported for patients with stage I disease. In the present treatment schedule we therefore differentiate between microscopic and macroscopic (grossly visible) tumor extension into the cervix.

The treatment of patients with microscopic tumor spread into the cervix is identical to that for patients with high risk stage I disease: primary hysterectomy and surgical staging. The indications and type of additional treatment are presented in figure 1.

The treatment of patients with macroscopic (grossly visible) tumor spread into the cervix justifies a different approach. Most commonly a combination of radiation i.e., preoperative external pelvic irradiation and/or intracavitary radium or cesium, followed in 4-6 weeks by total abdominal hysterectomy and bilateral salpingo-oophorectomy is performed. Preoperative radiation allows for optimal geometry of the intracavitary insertion and reduces the risk of bowel fixation in the pelvis.

However, since there is no convincing evidence of the value of preoperative radiation therapy, like for stage I disease, a more rational approach for stage II disease would be to perform primary surgery by means of a radical hysterectomy, surgical staging and individualized postoperative radiation on individualized basis, depending on the results of the surgical staging.

References

1. Pettersson F (ed.): Annual report on the results of treatment. In Gynaecologic Cancer. vol. 20, Stockholm, FIGO (1988)
2. Jones HW.: Treatment of adenocarcinoma of the endometrium. Obstet and Gynecol Survey 30: 147 (1975)
3. Aalders JG, Abeler V, Kolstad P, Onsrud M.: Postoperative external irradiation and prognostic parameters in stage I endometrial carcinoma. Obstet Gynecol 56: 419 (1980)
4. Lotocki RJ, Copeland LJ, De Petrillo AD, Muirhead W.: Stage I Endometrial adenocarcinoma: Treatment results in 835 patients. Am J Obstet Gynecol 146: 141 (1983)
5. Piver MS, Yazigi R, Blumenson L, Tsukada Y.: A prospective trial comparing hysterectomy, hysterectomy plus vaginal radium and uterine radium plus hysterectomy in stage I endometrial carcinoma. Obstet Gynecol 54: 85 (1979)
6. Truskett ID, Constable WC.: Management of carcinoma of the corporus uteri. Am J Obstet Gynecol 101: 689 (1968)
7. Potish RA, Twiggs LB, Adcock LL, Savage JE, Levitt SH, Prem KA.: Paraaortic lymph node radiotherapy in cancer of the uterine corpus. Obstet Gynecol 65: 251 (1985)
8. Creasman WT, DiSaia PJ, Blessin J, Wilkinson RH, Weed JC.: Prognostic significance of peritoneal cytology in patients with endometrial cancer and preliminary data concerning therapy with intraperitoneal radiopharmaceuticals. Am J Obstet Gynecol 141: 921 (1981)
9. Piver MS.: Progesterone therapy for malignant peritoneal cytology in surgical stage I endometrial adenocarcinoma. Seminars in Oncology 15 no.2 suppl.1: 50 (1988)
10. Lewis GC, Slack NH, Mortel R et al.: Adjuvant progestagen therapy in the primary definitive treatment of endometrial cancer. Gynecol Oncol 2: 368 (1974)
11. Vergote IBP, Kjorstad KE, Abeler V.: Randomized prospective trial of adjuvant progesterone in early endometrial cancer. In: Abstracts of the First Meeting of the International Gynecologic Cancer Society, Amsterdam (1987)

12. Kneale BG.: Adjuvant and therapeutic progestins in endometrial cancer. Clinics Obstet Gynaecol 13: 789 (1986)
13. Morrow CP, DiSaia PJ, Townsend DE.: Current management of endometrial carcinoma. Obstet Gynecol 42: 399 (1973)
14. Rutledge F.: The role of radical hysterectomy in adenocarcinoma of the endometrium. Gynecol Oncol 2: 331 (1974)
15. Onsrud M, Aalders JG, Abeler V, Taylor P.: Endometrial carcinoma with cervical involvement (stage II): prognostic factors and value of combined radiological-surgical treatment. Gynecol Oncol 13: 76 (1982)
16. Donavan JF.: Nonhormonal chemotherapy of endometrial adenocarcinoma. A review. Cancer 34: 1587 (1974)
17. Richard RM, Aalders JG, Bolonow RC, Morrow CP.: Endometrial cancer: state of the art. Contemporary Ob/Gyn 31 no. 6: 107 (1988)

IV. Radiotherapie

Postoperative Vaginal Irradiation by High-Dose-Rate Cobalt Afterloading in Stage I Endometrial Cancer: Experience from the Norwegian Radium Hospital

I. Vergote, K. Kjorstad, V. Abeler, and S. Vossli

Radiotherapy has been used in all its possible varieties as primary and adjuvant treatment of endometrial cancer. Still, the proper place of this treatment modality remains to be defined. Despite the large number of patients treated by a combination of surgery and radiotherapy, surprisingly there are no hard data showing improved survival in patients treated by radiotherapy [1,2]. However, adjuvant irradiation has been shown to reduce vaginal recurrences [2-4], and external pelvic irradiation decreases the risk of pelvic recurrences [5-7]. The prospective randomized trial, performed at The Norwegian Radium Hospital [5], showed clearly that external radiation therapy although decreasing local recurrence did not improve survival.

The first step in determining the role of radiotherapy is to search for a subset of patients treated with surgery only, and with a prognosis so good that adjuvant treatment is unwarranted. Since our treatment protocols in The Norwegian Radium Hospital prescribe some sort of radiotherapy to all patients with endometrial cancer, we had to go outside the Hospital to find such a material. With the help of The Norwegian Cancer Registry we were able to identify 305 patients with adenocarcinoma Stage I, treated with hysterectomy and bilateral adnexectomy only. These patients were not referred to a central institution, which would be the normal procedure in our country, mainly because of two reasons. Firstly, because the tumor infiltration was minimal, and secondly because the patient was too old or had a concomitant disease. All histological slides were reviewed by one of the authors. In retrospect the prognosis in relation to tumor grade is given in Table 1. It seems as if patients with highly differentiated tumors in Stage I would do very well with surgery alone. For Grade 2 and 3 tumors, the incidence of cancer deaths is so high that it cannot be argued that additional treatment would have been indicated if the patient's condition had allowed this. Vaginal vault recurrence carries a poor prognosis [2]. The incidence of vaginal top and suburethral recurrences in Stage I endometrial carcinoma ranges from 2-15% (mean 10%) [8]. Adjuvant vaginal radiation has resulted in a significant reduction in recurrence rate to 0,7-3% [2,3,9,10].

Table 1: Cause of death in 305 patients with endometrial cancer Stage I treated by surgery only.

Grade	n	Cause of death Cancer	Intercurrent disease
I	181	5 (3%)	20 (11%)
II	84	14 (17%)	16 (19%)
III	40	15 (38%)	4 (10%)
Total	305	34 (11%)	40 (13%)

Table 2: Relapse after surgery and vaginal high-dose Cobalt afterloading irradiation in low-risk* Stage I Endometrial cancer.

Group	None	Vaginal	Relapse Pelvis	Distant	Total
Grade 1	157	-	-	-	0/157
Grade 2	148	1	1	1	3/151
	305	1	1	1	3/308

*: Low risk: Grade 1 or 2, infiltration less than half of the myometrial thickness, adenocarcinoma, adenoacanthoma or adenosquamous adenocarcinoma

Table 3: Relapse after surgery and vaginal high-dose Cobalt afterloading irradiation in high-risk* Stage I Endometrial cancer.

Group	None	Vaginal	Relapse Pelvis	Distant	Total
Grade 1 + > 1/2#	15	-	-	1	1/16
Grade 2 + > 1/2#	32	-	2	1	3/35
Grade 3 + < 1/2	32	-	1	-	1/33
Grade 3 + > 1/2	4	-	2	1	3/7
Clear cell	9	1	3	1	5/14
	92	1	8	4	13/105

*: High-risk; Grade 3, or infiltration more than half of the myometrial thickness, or clear cell carcinoma.
#: infiltration more (>) or less (<) than half of the myometrial thickness

In The Norwegian Radium Hospital it has been the policy over the years to give vaginal irradiation to patients with low-risk Stage I endometrial cancer (Grade 1 or 2, infiltrating less than half of the myometrial thickness). In the sixties and seventies 25 mg of radium was inserted for 5 days, giving a dose of 3000 mgh to the vaginal top.

In 1978 we changed from radium to an afterloading high-dose rate Cobalt technique (Cathetron). This technique reduced the treatment time from days to minutes. The treatment can be given on an outpatient basis without the need for anesthetic or analgesic medication. One of the major advantages is the increased radiation protection for the medical personnel. The aim of the treatment was to give a dose to the vaginal mucosa equivalent to that delivered by the former continuous radium treatment. The dose was calculated to give the same CRE (Cumulated Radiation Effect) to a depth of 5 mm in the vaginal wall and was estimated to be 5,5 Gy per fraction, resulting in a total dose of 22 Gy in four fractions in the course of one week. The applicators used had diameters of 20, 25 and 30 mm. The largest possible applicator was used in order to distend the vaginal wall, thus securing optimal contact between the applicator and the target tissue. The cobalt source was longer than that used in the previous radium treatment. This way the whole vagina was irradiated instead of just the vaginal vault.

The inclusion criteria were the same as for the radium treatment (Stage I, Grade 1 or 2, infiltration less than half of the myometrial thickness). Some patients who did not meet the inclusion criteria, received vaginal Cathetron treatment instead of external irradiation, because of a bad general condition, high age, or other complicating diseases. After revision of all histological specimens by one of the authors, additional patients were found in whom the inclusion criteria had been violated. Recurrences were designated as vaginal, pelvic (without vaginal involvement), or distant (outside the lesser pelvis).

This high-dose rate Cobalt after-loading irradiation was given to 419 patients with Stage I endometrial cancer. At pathological review 6 patients had atypical adenomatous hyperplasia, resulting in 413 evaluable patients. After review, 308 patients had low-risk and 105 high-risk disease. The median follow-up is 54 months (range: 36-72 months). No patient is lost to follow-up. The median age is 60 years (range: 38-84 years).

Relapse rate and localization of relapse are presented in Table 2 and 3. Vaginal recurrence was seen in only 1 patient of the low-risk group (0,3%)

and 1 patient of the high-risk group (1%). Both patients died of their disease. In the entire material no suburethral recurrences were observed. In the total series 12 (2,9%) patients died of their disease and 11 (2,6%) of intercurrent disease.

Two hundred patients were interviewed according to a standardized questionnaire. The questionnaire concentrated on late radiation side effects. Only 2 patients (1%) claimed vaginal discomfort following the treatment. One of these patients had severe atrophy and agglutination of the vagina compatible with postirradiation damage. The other complained of itching and burning, but no objective symptoms of radiation damage could be found. Mandell et al [9], and Sorbe and Smeds [10] suggested that the incidence of vaginal complications is related to the dose per fraction. The low frequency of vaginal discomfort in this series can be explained by the relatively low dose per fraction (5,5 Gy) compared with the other studies using high-dose rate Cobalt vaginal irradiation [9,10].

As the intention of the treatment was to prevent vaginal recurrences in patients operated for endometrial cancer, the results are of course very satisfying. The question is how many patients have been treated unnecessarily. Better prognostic variables can possibly help us in the future to select the patients more accurately.

References

1. Jones HW III: Treatment of adenocarcinoma of the endometrium. Obstet Gynecol Survey 30: 147, 1975
2. Berek JS, Hacker NF, Hatch KD, Young RC: Uterine corpus and cervical cancer, Curr Probl Cancer 12: 65, 1988
3. Lotocki RJ, Copeland IJ, DePetrillo AD et al: Stage I endometrial adenocarcinoma: Treatment results in 835 patients. Am J Obstet Gynecol 146: 141, 1983
4. Reddy S, Lee Ms, Hendrickson FR: Pattern of recurrences in endometrial cancer and their management. Radiology 133: 737, 1979
5. Onsrud M, Kolstad P, Normann T: Postoperative external pelvic irradiation in carcinoma of the corpus Stage I: A controlled clinical trial. Gynecol Oncol 4: 222-231, 1976
6. Salazar OM, Feldstein ML, DePapp EW et al: Endometrial carcinoma: Analysis of failures with special emphasis on the use of initial preoperative external pelvic irradiation. Int J Radiat Oncol Biol Phys 2: 1101, 1977

7. Kucera H, Vavra N, Weghaupt K: Benefit of external irradiation in pathologic Stage I endometrial carcinoma: A prospective clinical trial of 605 patients who received postoperative vaginal irradiation and additional pelvic irradiation in the presence of unfavorable prognostic factors. Gynecol Oncol 38: 99, 1990
8. Leibel SA, Wharam MD: Vaginal and para-aortic lymph node metastases in carcinoma of the endometrium. Int J Radiat Oncol Biol Phys 6: 893-914, 1980
9. Mandell L, Dattatreyudu N, Anderson L, Hilaris B: Postoperative vaginal radiation in endometrial cancer using remote afterloading technique. Int J Radiat Oncol Biol Phys 11: 473, 1985
10. Sorbe B, Smeds AC: Postoperative vaginal irradiation by a high dose rate afterloading technique in endometrial carcinoma Stage I. Acta Oncol 28: 679, 1989

V. Hormontherapie

Adjuvante Hormontherapie beim Endometriumkarzinom

Manfred Kaufmann

Das in westlichen Ländern häufige Endometriumkarzinom hat im allgemeinen eine recht günstige Prognose. Bei diesem grundsätzlich hormonabhängigen Tumor rezidivieren dennoch ein Drittel der Patientinnen nach Primärbehandlung und werden an dieser Erkrankung sterben. Lt. der 20. Ausgabe [9] des FIGO-Reports (Int. Fed. of Gyn. and Obstr.) liegen die Fünf-Jahres-Überlebensdaten beim Stadium I bei 72,3% (11.035 Patienten), beim Stadium II bei 56,4% (1.135 Patienten). Die Heilungschancen und das Überleben sind dabei wesentlich von bestimmten Risikofaktoren (Diabetes, Adipositas, Hypertonie) und Prognosefaktoren (Tumorstadium, Differenzierungsgrad des Tumors, myometrane Infiltrationstiefe, Spülcytologie des Peritoneums, Hormonrezeptorstatus, Ploidiegrad, S-Phasen-Anteil, Onkogenamplifikation) abhängig.

Eine wesentliche Verbesserung der bisher erzielten Therapieergebnisse läßt sich neben der Prävention durch eine bessere Früherkennung, bessere Staging-Verfahren sowie durch die Anwendung verläßlicherer Prognosefaktoren [5] derzeit wohl nur durch den Einsatz systemischer adjuvanter Therapieverfahren erzielen. Hormontherapien wurden bisher beim rezidivierten und fernmetastasierten Korpuskarzinom erfolgreich eingesetzt [11,12].

Die Ergebnisse verschiedener Pilotuntersuchungen hinsichtlich der Wirksamkeit adjuvanter Hormontherapien, insbesondere von Gestagentherapien, haben beim Endometriumkarzinom bisher sehr widersprüchliche Ergebnisse gezeigt. Es bestehen insbesondere auch nur lückenhafte Informationen über einen möglichen therapeutischen Gewinn in Relation zu therapieinduzierten Nebenwirkungen. Vor allem sind bisher nicht genau definierte Patientenkollektive adjuvant therapiert und analysiert worden.

Im folgenden sollen deshalb zwei prospektiv durchgeführte randomisierte Untersuchungen mit ausreichend großen Patientenkollektiven berichtet und kommentiert werden.

Ziel einer am norwegischen Radium-Hospital von 1/1975-6/1982 bei 1.148 Patienten durchgeführten Studie [13] war, ob eine adjuvante Progestagentherapie beim Endometriumkarzinom des Stadiums FIGO I und II das Überleben verbessert. In dieser zweiarmigen Studie wurde ein Kontrollarm ohne weitere postoperative adjuvante systemische Therapie mit dem Therapiearm verglichen. Die lokale primäre Therapiestrategie war neben der Hysterektomie und beidseitiger Adnexektomie eine externe Bestrahlung des kleinen Beckens, welche bei Tumoren mit einer Infiltration über 1/2 des Myometriums oder bei einem Grad III angewandt wurde. Sonst erhielten die Patientinnen eine vaginale Auslastung. Frauen mit einem Stadium II wurden präoperativ mit intracavitärer Radiumapplikation behandelt.

Die Behandlungsgruppe erhielt 1-6 Wochen postoperativ zunächst eine Loading-Dosis von 5.000 mg Hydroxyprogesteroncaproat über 5 Tage und anschließend dieses Hormon 2 x wöchentlich i.m. über ein Jahr mit einer Dosierung von 1.000 mg. Die mediane Nachbeobachtungszeit betrug 72 Monate (42-132). Auswertbar waren 531 Patientinnen der Kontrollgruppe und 553 Patientinnen der Progestagen-Gruppe. Das mittlere Alter der Patientinnen betrug 61 Jahre.

Eine Gleichverteilung von verschiedenen Prognosefaktoren war in beiden Patientenkollektiven gegeben (Anteil von Adenokarzinomen ca. 87%, gut differenzierte Tumoren ca. 41%, keine Myometrane Infiltration ca. 13%, operativ-pathologisches Stadium I ca. 90% und Stadium II ca. 10%).

Zwischen der Therapie- und Kontrollgruppe zeigten die unbereinigten Daten keinen Unterschied hinsichtlich der Überlebensraten (Abb. 1). Dies galt auch für tumorbedingte Todesfälle. In der Therapiegruppe wurde eine signifikant höhere Todesrate aufgrund von Sekundärerkrankungen festgestellt (p=0,04). Das mediane Überleben von Patientinnen mit krebsbedingter Todesursache war in der Therapiegruppe im Vergleich zur Kontrollgruppe (30 versus 22 Monate) signifikant (p=0,03) günstiger. Die Rezidivrate unterschied sich in beiden Gruppen nicht (67 Frauen in der Therapiegruppe versus 75 Patientinnen in der Kontrollgruppe); ebenso wenig das rezidivfreie Intervall (20 versus 17 Monate). Es ergab sich auch kein Unterschied für die verschiedenen Karzinomtypen. Insgesamt zeigten aber Frauen mit einem Adenokarzinom und einem Differenzierungsgrad II bzw. einer Myometriuminfiltration über die Hälfte unter der Therapie weniger Rezidive im Vergleich zur Kontrollgruppe. Rezidive waren im Beckenbereich in beiden Kollektiven gleich häufig. Adjuvant therapierte Frauen zeigten jedoch weniger Fernmetastasen (25 versus 35 Patienten).

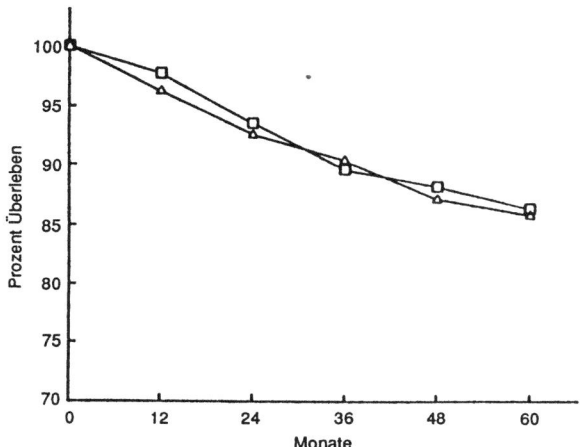

Abb. 1: Gesamtüberleben bei 553 Patientinnen mit einjähriger adjuvanter Hydroxyprogesteroncaproattherapie versus 531 Kontrollpatienten [nach 13]
■ = Therapiegruppe / △ = Kontrollgruppe

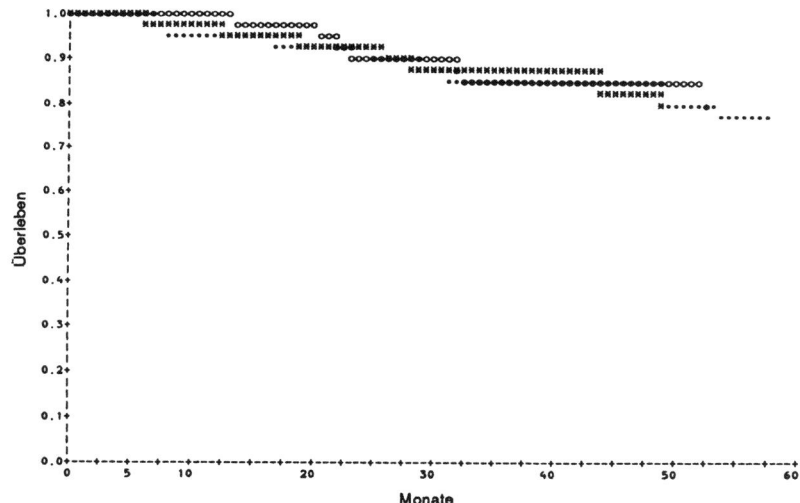

Abb. 2: Gesamtüberleben [life table analysis nach 2] von 385 Patienten mit Endometriumkarzinom Stadium I FIGO und adjuvanter Hormontherapie (Kontrolle versus Tamoxifen versus Medroxyprogesteronacetat) [nach 3]
** = Kontrolle / ooo = Tamoxifen / ... = Medroxyprogesteronacetat

461 sog. high-risk-Patientinnen [nach 4] (Grad III Adenokarzinom oder Adenokarzinom mit Infiltration der äußeren 2/3 des Myometriums oder Adenokarzinom des Stadiums II oder III oder adenosquamöses Karzinom, Klarzellkarzinom, seröses oder undifferenziertes Karzinom) zeigten trendmäßig weniger krebsbedingte Todesfälle und ein besseres rezidivfreies Überleben bei adjuvanter Behandlung; das Gesamtüberleben blieb jedoch unbeeinflußt. 233 Frauen erhielten eine Progestagentherapie und 228 Frauen dienten als Kontrollgruppe. 66 Frauen starben in der Therapie- und 64 Frauen in der Kontrollgruppe. Karzinombedingte Todesfälle waren in der Therapiegruppe weniger im Vergleich zur Kontrollgruppe (39 versus 50, p=0,68). Allerdings starben mehr Frauen an Sekundärerkrankungen in der Therapiegruppe (27 versus 14, p=0,09). In der Therapiegruppe wurden 44 und in der Kontrollgruppe 58 Rezidive (p=0,11) beobachtet. Die Fünf-Jahres-Überlebensrate betrug 82% in der Therapie- und 75% in der Kontrollgruppe (p=0,1).

Im Rahmen einer südwestdeutschen Studiengruppe [3] wurde zwischen 4/1983 und 10/1989 bei 385 Patienten eine dreiarmige, prospektiv randomisierte Studie beim Stadium FIGO I des Endometriumkarzinoms durchgeführt. Ziel dieser Studie war die Wirkung verschiedener adjuvanter endokriner Therapien hinsichtlich des Überlebens und der Toxizität im Vergleich zu einer Kontrollgruppe zu untersuchen. Bei allen Frauen wurde eine abdominale Hysterektomie mit beidseitiger Adnexektomie unter Mitnahme einer Scheidenmanschette und meist einer intravaginalen Kontakttherapie durchgeführt. Eine Bestrahlung des kleinen Beckens erfolgte bei Grad-III-Karzinomen oder bei einer myometranen Invasion mehr als 1/3 der Myometrium-Gesamtdicke. Die mediane Nachbeobachtungszeit betrug 31 Monate. In je einem Therapiearm wurden Tamoxifen (30 mg) als Antiöstrogen oder Medroxyprogesteronacetat (500 mg) als Gestagen für jeweils 2 Jahre per os gegeben.

66,7% der Frauen waren 51-70 Jahre alt, nur 6,8% jünger als 50 und 26,5% älter als 70 Jahre. 48,8% der Tumoren wurden als Grad I, 40,5% als Grad II und 10,7% als Grad III-Tumoren eingestuft.

Das Gesamtüberleben des Gesamtkollektives war für Frauen jünger als 70 Jahre signifikant (p<0,001) besser; ebenfalls für Grad I/II-Tumoren im Vergleich zu Grad III-Tumoren (p<0,0001). In der Kontrollgruppe wurden 8,8% Rezidive beobachtet im Vergleich zu 10,9% in der mit Tamoxifen (Tam) behandelten Gruppe und 7,4% in der mit Medroxyprogesteronacetat (MPA) behandelten Gruppe. Die wenigsten Lokalrezidive wurden unter

Tabelle 1: Wirkung der adjuvanten Hormontherapie auf die Rezidivhäufigkeit und das Überleben beim Endometriumkarzinom Stadium I FIGO

	No. (%) Kontrolle n=135	Tamoxifen (TAM) n=128	Medroxyprogesteron-acetat (MPA) n=122
Lokalrezidiv	5 (3,7)	2 (1,6)	5 (4,1)
Fernmetastasen	6 (4,4)	9 (7,0)	4 (3,3)
Beides	1 (0,7)	3 (2,3)	0 (0)
Todesfälle	14 (10,4)	12 (9,4)	17 (13,9)

Tabelle 2: Nebenwirkungen der adjuvanten Hormontherapie beim Endometriumkarzinom Stadium I FIGO

Hauptnebenwirkungen	Anzahl der Patienten		
	Kontrolle	TAM	MPA
Gewichtszunahme	4	5	18
Flüssigkeitseinlagerung	1	2	6
Übelkeit/Erbrechen	1	4	3
Thrombose	1	1	1
Lungenembolie	0	0	1
Hitzewallungen	1	12	4
Muskelkrämpfe	0	1	5
trockene Haut	0	2	0
Dekompensation Hypertonie	2	2	0
" Diabetes mell.	3	0	1
" Kardial	1	0	1
psychische Veränderungen	0	0	1
andere	7	3	6
Gesamt:	21	32	47

Tamoxifen und die wenigsten Fernmetastasen unter Medroxyprogesteronacetat beobachtet (Tabelle 1). Die Anzahl verstorbener Frauen war in der Medroxyprogesteronacetat-Therapiegruppe mit 13,9% im Vergleich zur Kontrollgruppe (10,4%) und der Tamoxifen-Therapiegruppe (9,4%) am höchsten. Abbildung 2 zeigt das Gesamtüberleben der 385 Patientinnen für alle drei Kollektive. Es ergaben sich keine signifikanten Unterschiede zwischen den einzelnen Therapiegruppen.

Die wichtisten registrierten Nebenwirkungen und beobachteten Begleiterkrankungen sind für alle drei Therapiearme in Tabelle 2 dargestellt. Es zeigte sich, daß die meisten Nebenwirkungen durch Medroxyprogesteronacetat hervorgerufen wurden. Am häufigsten wurde hier eine Gewichtszunahme registriert und als schwerste Nebenwirkung je eine Thrombose und eine Lungenembolie beobachtet.

Ergebnisse verschiedener historischer Untersuchungen bzw. von Pilotstudien legten die Vermutung nahe, daß eine adjuvante Gestagentherapie die Rezidivrate verringern und gleichzeitig auch das Überleben des Endometriumkarzinoms im frühen Stadium verlängern können. Bisher berichtete prospektiv randomisierte Studien [1,6,7,8] im Zeitraum 1974 bis 1988 lassen allerdings keinen Nutzen einer adjuvanten Therapie mit Progestagenen erkennen. Allerdings sind diese Studien in ihrer Aussagekraft begrenzt, da einerseits entweder eine zu geringe Anzahl an Patienten untersucht wurde, die Nachbeobachtungszeiten zu kurz oder zu viele Patientinnen nach einer Randomisation nicht mehr auswertbar waren.

Die beiden vorgestellten Studien [3,13] weisen einerseits ausreichend große Patientenzahlen und andererseits eine entsprechend lange Nachbeobachtungszeit auf. In beiden Untersuchungen läßt sich keine Verbesserung der Gesamtüberlebensrate durch eine adjuvante, i.m. applizierte Medroxyprogesteroncaproattherapie, eine orale Medroxyprogesteronacetattherapie oder eine Antiöstrogentherapie mit Tamoxifen aufzeigen. Signifikante Unterschiede hinsichtlich der Rezidivrate bzw. ein signifikanter Unterschied in der Mortalität aufgrund des Endometriumkarzinoms lassen sich ebenfalls nicht erkennen. Damit sind die bisher vorliegenden Ergebnisse zur adjuvanten Hormontherapie beim Endometriumkarzinom eher enttäuschend. Die geringen objektiven Ansprechraten gegenüber den in verschiedenen Untersuchungen genannten Ansprechraten von ca. 1/3 aller Fälle lassen erkennen, daß sich in der adjuvanten Situation die erwartete Effektivität nicht aufzeigen läßt. Ursache dafür mag eine sehr unterschiedliche geringere Hormonsensitivität der verschiedenen Tumortypen sein. Der Nachweis von Hormonrezeptoren scheint hier wenig aussagekräftig.

Verläßlichere Prognosefaktoren sollten deshalb gefunden werden. Andererseits scheint eine Hormonabhängigkeit vor allem bei prognostisch günstigem Grading vorzuliegen, so daß Patientinnen mit ungünstiger Prognose von adjuvanten hormonellen Therapiemaßnahmen nicht profitieren. Erste in-vitro-Untersuchungen lassen beispielsweise die klinisch bekannte Chemoresistenz beim Endometriumkarzinom nachweisen [10]. Über den Nachweis von P-170-Glykoprotein in der Zellmembran gelang es, Informationen über die sog. multiple drug resistance zu erhalten. In allen bisher untersuchten Fällen war eine solche Resistenz vorhanden, damit scheint auch eine cytotoxische adjuvante Therapie wenig erfolgversprechend. Einzelne adjuvante cytotoxische Therapiestudien scheinen dies zu bestätigen.

Zukünftige prospektive randomisierte Studien sollten deshalb in verschiedenen prognostisch definierten Subgruppen mit z.B. ungünstiger Prognose (High-Risk-Situation) weiter den Nutzen einer adjuvanten Hormon- bzw. cytotoxischen Therapie untersuchen. Bekanntermaßen finden sich u.a. bei Patientinnen mit Korpuskarzinom verschiedene klinische Risikofaktoren bzw. Begleiterkrankungen, welche günstig bzw. auch ungünstig durch eine systemische Hormontherapie beeinflußt werden können, was in den beiden berichteten Studien beobachtet wurde. Es muß dabei insbesondere berücksichtigt werden, daß therapieinduzierte, nicht karzinombedingte Todesfälle unter derartigen Therapien zunehmen können. Inwieweit beispielsweise durch eine adjuvante Antiöstrogentherapie die Rate kardiovasculärer Erkrankungen reduziert werden kann, bleibt ebenfalls weiteren Analysen vorbehalten.

Literatur:

1. De Palo G, Mersom M, Del Vecchio M et al: A controlled clinical study of adjuvant medroxyprogesterone acetate (MPA) therapy in pathological stage I endometrial cancer with myometrial invasion (Abstr.). Proc. Am. Soc. Clin. Oncol. 4: 121 (1985)
2. Kaplan EL, Meier P: Non-parametric estimation from incomplete observation. J. Am. Statist. Assoc. 53: 457-481 (1958)
3. Kaufmann M, Abel U, Brunnert K, Kreienberg R, Melchert F, Mösch R, Neises M, Scherman J, Schmid H, Seeger F, Seufert R, Staiger HF, Stiglmeyer R, and Stosiek U for the South West Gynecological Oncology Group (SWGGOG): Adjuvant treatment with Tamoxifen (TAM) od Medroxyprogesterone Acetate (MPA) or Observation only in pathological

Stage I endometrial carcinoma. In: Adjuvant Therapy of Cancer VI. SE Salmon (Edt.) WB Saunders Company Philadelphia 1990 pp. 522-526
4. Kneale BLG: Adjunctive and therapeutic progestins in endometrial cancer. Clin. Obstet Gynaecol 13: 789-809 (1986)
5. Kühn W, Kaufmann M, Feichter GE, Rummel HH, Abel U, Heep J, v.Minckwitz G: Prognostische Bedeutung zellkinetischer Parameter beim Endometriumkarzinom. Geburtsh. u. Frauenheilk. 49: 787-792 (1989)
6. Lewis GC, Nelson HS, Mortel R, Bross D: Adjuvant progestagen therapy in the primary definitive treatment of endometrial cancer. Gynecol. Oncol. 2: 368-376 (1974)
7. Macdonald RR, Thorogood J, Mason M: A randomized trial of progestagens in the primary treatment of endometrial cancer. Br J Obstet Gynaecol 95: 166-174 (1988)
8. Malkasian GD, Decker DG: Adjuvant progesterone therapy for stage I endometrial carcinoma. Int J Gynaecol Obstet 16: 48-49 (1978)
9. Pettersson F (ed): Annual Report on the results of treatment in gynecological cancer. 20th Edt. FIGO Stockholm, 1989
10. Schneider J, Efferth T, Kaufmann M, Matia JC, Mattern J, Rodriguez-Escudero FJ, Volm M: Expression of the multidrug-resistance gene product P-glycoprotein in gynecological tumors. The Cancer Journal 3: 202-205 (1990)
11. Schulz KD, Rück A, Zippel HH et al: Endometrial Cancer. Advances in Clinical Oncology 3: 95-110 (1988)
12. Thigpen T: Systemic therapy with single agents for advanced or recurrent endometrial carcinoma. In: Surwit EA, Alberts DS (edts): Endometrial cancer. Kluwer Academic Pub Boston, Dordrecht, London, 93-106, 1989
13. Vergote J, Kjorstad K, Abeler V, Kolstad P: A randomized trial of adjuvant progestagen in early endometrial cancer. Cancer 64: 1011-1016 (1989)

Palliative Hormonal Treatment in Endometrial Carcinoma*

K.-D. Schulz, J. Hofmann, R. Hackenberg,
G. Emons, P. Schmidt-Rhode, and G. Sturm

At first sight the description of the palliative hormonal treatment methods in disseminated malignant endometrial tumors is a simple exercise requiring only a few minutes. This anticipation is true if only the presently established therapeutic models are described.

1. Present status of the art

The growth control of hormone-dependent endometrial carcinoma by oestrogens and progesterone is a well known fact since decades. The intracellular interaction between both hormones is fundamentel for the actual therapeutic strageties (Fig.1). Since the late fifties and early sixties progestogens are commonly used to antagonize the oestrogen-dependent tumor cell proliferation [1,2]. Progestogens are capable of inhibiting the growth of endometrial carcinoma in nearly 30% of all cases without severe side effects. The clinical experiences were obtained using different progestational compounds in thousands of patients [reviewed by 3]. The first step of the oestrogen-antagonizing effect of progestogens includes alterations at the steroid receptor level; the synthesis of oestrogen receptors is inhibited and the biological inactivation of intracellular oestrogens is increased [reviewed by 4] by the induction of oestrogen metabolizing enzymes.

---

* The own investigations were supported by the »Deutsche Forschungsgemeinschaft« (Schu 631/1-1)
** dedicated to Prof. Dr. med. Klaus Thomsen, past director of the Department of Obstetrics and Gynecology, University of Hamburg, on the occasion of his 75th birthday

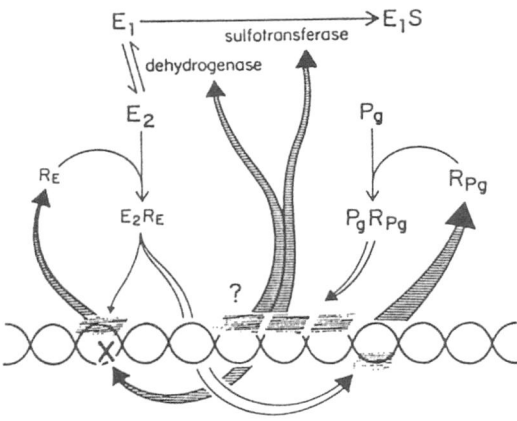

Fig.1: Intracellular interaction for oestrogens and progesterone in normal endometrial cells and in hormone-dependent endometrial carcinoma [4]

R_E = oestrogen receptor E_2R_E = oestrogen receptor complex

E_1 = oestrone E_2 = oestradiol

E_1S = oestrone sulfate R_{pg} = progesterone receptor

PgR_{pg} = progesterone receptor complex   p = progesterone

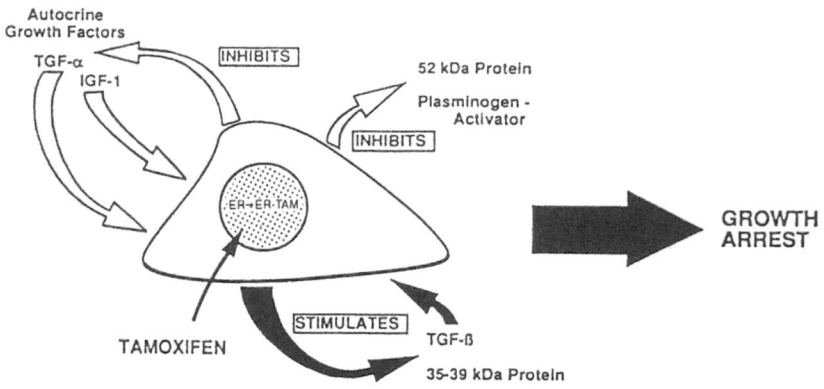

Fig.2: The inhibition of oestrogen-stimulated growth in breast cancer cells by tamoxifen [10]

Alterations of the hormonal tumor-host-balance are of additional significance [5,6,7,8], but preferentially following the administration of high dose progestogens. Beside progestogens other substances counteracting the effect of oestrogens might be recommended, i.e. antioestrogens and aromatase inhibitors. Only small clinical experiences are existent using the antioestrogen tamoxifen. Analyzing the efficacy in 116 unselected cases of disseminated tumors [9], an overall response of 26% has been reported. The action of tamoxifen in endometrial cancer cells might be very similar to observations made in hormone-dependent breast cancer (Fig.2) [summarized by 10]. Presently however, this supposition has to be submitted urgently to proof. Fig. 3 and 4 show [11], that tamoxifen effects on the concentration of circulating hormones are relatively small in ovarectomized or postmenopausal women. They are presumably of minor relevance for the inhibition of tumor cell proliferation. The present selection criteria for the application of antioestrogens are very similar to those employed for progestogens. Doses between 20 and 40 mg/day do not demonstrate an unequivocal efficacy.

The usefulness of aromatase inhibitors is more speculative today. Using aminoglutethimide, a response rate of 22% has been published in a pilot study [12]. Therefore the routine use of aromatase inhibitors cannot be recommended. If indicated, daily oral doses of 500 or 1000 mg aminoglutethimide should be given combined with a corticosteroid replacement therapy. The mode of action seems to be comparable with observations obtained in breast cancer (Fig.5) [13].

We are aware of the controversially discussed recommendation to use tamoxifen as second line treatment. Recently a very small patient group has been reported showing no response to tamoxifen after a preceding progestogen therapy.

On the other hand the present informations about the efficacy of tamoxifen as primary therapy are extremely limited. Hitherto the correlation of the possible tumor response to morphological or biochemical selection criteria has not been proven sufficiently. In our opinion it is to early to recommend generally the replacement of progestogens by antioestrogens as first line treatment. Additionally one should keep in mind the small, but distinct oestrogen-like effects of the antioestrogenic compounds presently used. Therefore the primary administration of tamoxifen should be restricted to patients showing varying contraindications for the use of progestogens.

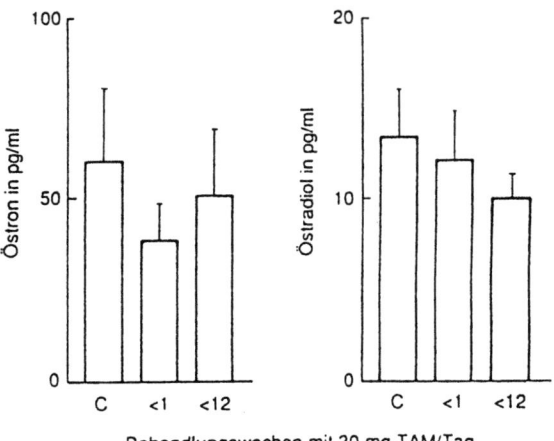

Fig.3: Plasma concentrations oestrone and oestradiol in postmenopausal patients under continuous treatment with 30 mg tamoxifen/day [11]

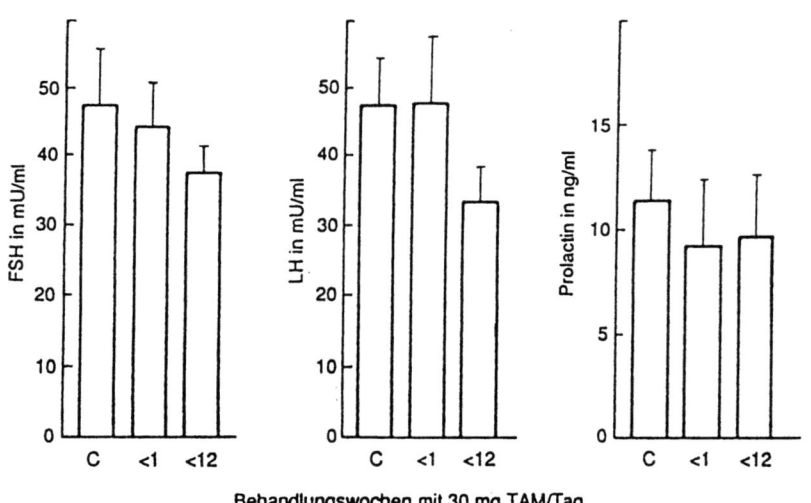

Fig.4: FSH-, LH- and prolactin plasma concentrations in postmenopausal patients under continuous treatment with 30 mg tamoxifen/day [11]

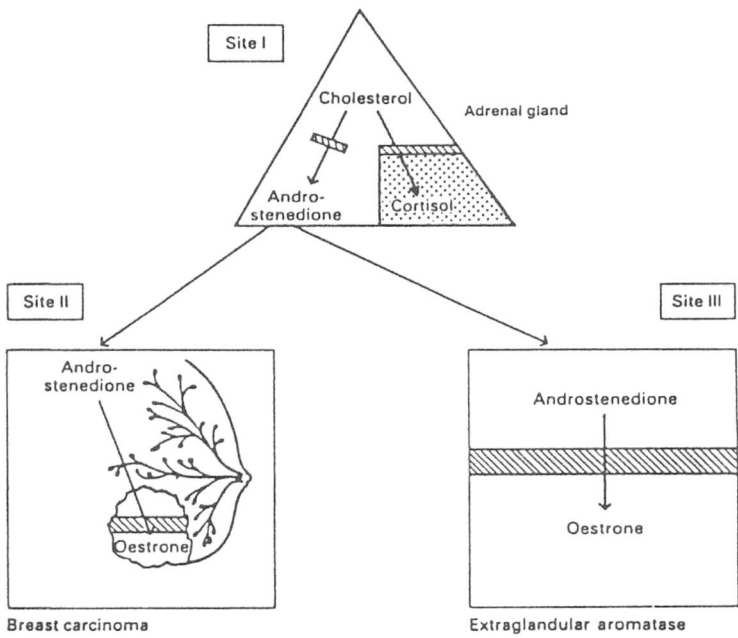

Fig.5: Multilateral blockade of oestrogens-synthesis by the aromatase inhibitor aminoglutethimide in breast cancer patients [13]

2. How to improve present endocrine treatment methods?

Up to now all efforts are centralized to the interaction between oestrogens and progestins. The chance for the development of new treatment modalities on this field is relatively low. This opinion is supported by disappointing observations previously made. Highly promising combinations of antioestrogens and progestogens or progestogens and polychemotherapy did not fulfill the expectations up to now.

The current discussion of low dose or <u>high dose progestogen therapy</u> brings possibly a partial advantage to a limited risk group of endometrial carcinoma patients.

Table 1: Summarized published cases of disseminated endometrial carcinoma under »low« and »high dose« treatment with medroxyprogesterone acetate [adapted to reviews 15,16,17]

	number of patients	% responder (CR and PR)
high dose MPA-therapy (>100 ng MPA/ml plasma)	273	45
low dose MPA-therapy (<100 ng MPA/ml plasma)	156	31

Table 2: High dose medroxyprogesterone acetate therapy in disseminated endometrial carcinoma dependent on dose and morphological grading [20]

Dose i.m./week	G1		G3	
	n.	response %	n.	response %
500 mg	15	40,0	11	18,2
1000 mg	79	54,4	25	36,0
2 x 1000 mg	19	57,9	8	37,5

While low doses of different progestogen exert their tumor inhibiting effects preferentially on the cellular level, high doses develop general endocrine effects in the whole organism influencing additionally the growth of hormone-dependent endometrial malignancies. The best and most detailed informations are available for Medroxyprogesterone acetate (MPA) [5,6,7,8].

The table 1 summarizes patients with disseminated endometrial cancer published in the literature and treated with different doses of MPA [reviewed by 15,16,17]. The detailed description of the treatment methods used, allowed the pharmacokinetic association with the high and low dose principle. While high dose regimen induced generally a remission rate of

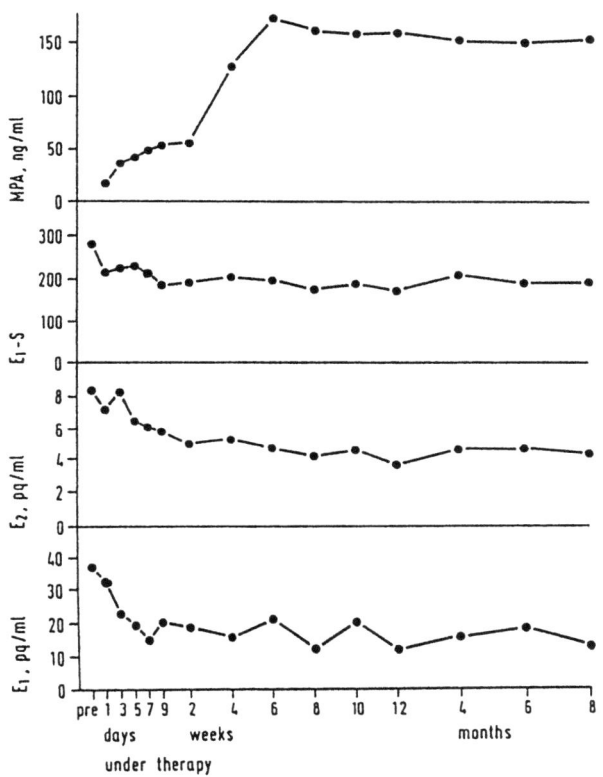

Fig.6: Circulating oestrogens under oral high dose MPA therapy (1000 mg/day) in postmenopausal breast cancer patients [7,14]

45% in unselected cases, the low dose progestogen therapy was only effective in about 30% of patients. Tab. 2 shows, that intramuscular doses of 1000 mg or 2000 mg per week increase generally the response rate in advanced endometrial tumors, but predominantly in poorly differentiated cancers [20]. According to pharmacokinetic findings the described dose corresponds nearly completely with the oral high dose MPA-therapy of 1000 mg daily [7,14]. The high dose regimen leads to MPA plasma concentration of 100 ng/ml and more, being necessary to reduce circulating

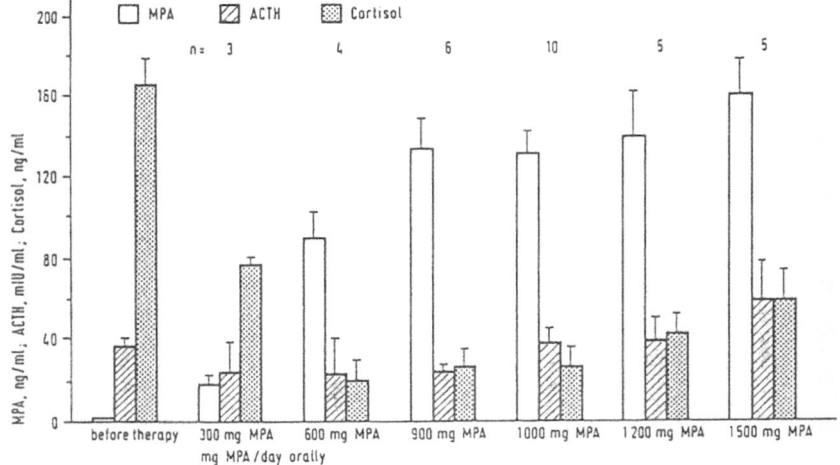

Fig.7: The influence of different continuous oral doses of medroxyprogesterone acetate (MPA) on plasma concentrations of MPA, ACTH and cortisol in postmenopausal breast cancer patients [7,14]

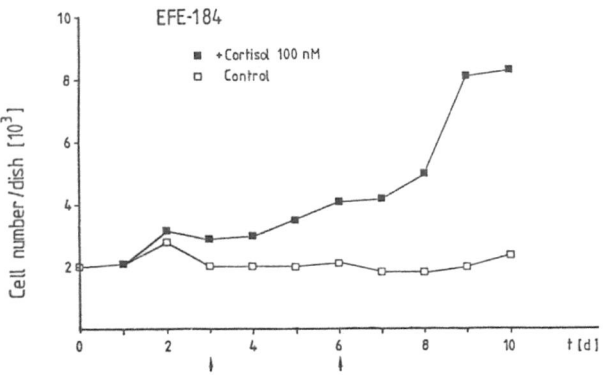

Fig.8: In vitro effects of cortisol on the proliferation of an oestrogen-independent human endometrial carcinoma cell line [19]

oestrogens in postmenopausal women (Fig. 6) and to suppress adrenal corticosteroids synthesis (Fig. 7) [7]. But how to explain the clear clinical efficacy of high dose MPA in poorly differentiated, mostly oestrogen-independent corpus neoplasia? Some authors believe, that very high MPA plasma concentrations develop receptor independent cytotoxic actions. But this supposition does not agree with observations obtained in in vitro models showing no influence of 10^{-6}M MPA on the cell proliferation [18]. Another explanation might be given by an individual, oestrogen-independent human endometrial cancer cell line. As published recently [19], this cell line contained relatively high concentrations of corticosteroid receptors. Cortisol increase significantly the cell proliferation of this tumor type in vitro (Fig. 8). The deprivation of endogeneous corticosteroids in vivo by high dose MPA might explain the unexpected inhibition of some oestrogen-independent, high-risk endometrial cancers.

Summarizing these experiences, we prefer in the meantime a more graded management of the gestagen application. In highly differentiated G1-tumors showing a specific progesterone binding of more than 100 fmol/mg tumor protein, daily oral doses of 200-300 mg MPA are sufficient. But in tumors with marginal hormone-dependence and with presumable functional heterogeneity, characterized by a G2-grading and by a relatively low binding of progesterone between 50 to 100 fmol/mg tumor protein, daily MPA-doses have to be elevated to 1000 mg. Balancing the efficacy and the side effects, the high dose principle might be useful too in selected single high risk tumors, replacing there an intolerable, aggresive polychemotherapy.

This additional therapeutic chance is of large clinical relevance as some authors reported the progredient loss of progesterone receptors, i.e. the loss of hormone sensitivity, in disseminate and recurrent tumors.

References

1. Kaiser R: Die Wirkung von Gestagenen beim Korpuskarzinom. Arch. Gynaek. 193: 195, 1959
2. Kelley RM, Baker WH: Progestational agents in the treatment of carcinoma of the endometrium. New Engl. J. Med. 264: 216, 1961
3. Richardson GS, Mac Laughlin DT: Hormonal biology of endometrial cancer. UICC Technical Report Series 42, 1978

4. Brooks SC, Christensen C, Meyers S, Corombos J, Pack BA: Endocrine implications of endometrial estrogen sulfurylation. In: »Steroids and endometrial cancer«. Jasonni VM, Nenci J, Flamigni C (eds). Raven Press, New York, p. 145, 1983
5. Pannuti F, Giovannini M, Martoni A, Fruet F, Rubino J, Vecchi F, Zanichelli L, Pieromaldi S: Effects of high dose oral medroxyprogesterone acetate (MPA) on plasma levels of T3, T4, TSH, LH, FSH, PRL, 17ß-oestradiol, testosterone and aldosterone. IRCS Med. Sci, 8: 764, 1980
6. Pannuti F, Martoni A, Camaggi CM et al: High dose medroxyprogesterone acetate in oncology: history, clinical use and pharmacokinetics. In: »Int. Symp. Medroxy progesterone Acetate«. Cavalli F et al (eds), Excerpta Medica, p. 5, 1982
7. Schulz KD, Schmidt-Rhode P, Sturm G: High dose medroxyprogesterone acetate in breast cancer-present state of knowledge. In: »Progress in hormono- and chemotherapy«. Robustelli della Cuna G, Nagel GA, Lanius,P (eds) Kehrer, Freiburg, p. 21, 1985
8. Schulz KD, Schmidt-Rhode P, Zippel HH, Sturm G: New Concepts of Adjuvant Drug Treatment in Endometrial Cancer. In: »Endometrial Cancer«. Schulz KD, King RJB, Pollow K, Taylor RW (eds), Zuckschwerdt, München, p. 169, 1987
9. Swenerton KD: Antioestrogens for the treatment of endometrial cancer. In: »Endometrial Cancer«. Schulz K-D, King RJB, Pollow K, Taylor RW (eds), Zuckschwerdt, München, p. 165, 1987
10. Jordan VC: Resistance to antioestrogen therapy: a challenge for the future. In: Cavalli F (Ed): Endocrine therapy of breast cancer III. Springer Berlin, p. 51-60, 1989
11. Schulz KD, Sturm G, Schmidt-Rhode P, Hackenberg R, Künzig HJ: Pharmakokinetik und Pharmakodynamik der Antiöstrogene. In: Kubli F et al (Eds): Neue Wege in der Brustkrebsbehandlung. Zuckschwerdt München, p. 62, 1983
12. Murray RML, Pitt P: Treatment of advanced metastatic breast cancer, carcinoma of the prostate and endometrial cancer with aminoglutethimide. In: »Aminoglutethimide as an aromatase inhibitor in the treatment of cancer«. Nagel GA, Santen RJ (eds) Hans Huber Publishers Bern, p. 109, 1984
13. Santen RJ, Lipton A, Harvey H, Boucher AE, Henderson C: Pharmacological mechanisms of oestrogen Suppression with aminoglutethimide in women with breast cancer. In: »Aminoglutethimide as an aromatase inhibitor in the treatment of cancer«. Nagel GA, Santen RJ (eds), Hans Huber Publishers Bern, p. 38, 1984
14. Schulz KD, Rück A, Zippel HH, Hofmann J, Hackenberg R, Schmidt-Rhode P, Hölzel F, Pfisterer Y: Endometrial Cancer, Advances in Clinical Oncology 3: 95, 1988

15. Bonte J, Decoster MJ, Ide P, Billiet G: Hormonoprophylaxis and Hormonotherapy in the treatment of Endometrial Adenocarcinoma by means of Medroxyprogesterone Acetate. Gynecol. Oncol. 6: 60, 1978
16. Bonte J. Hormone dependency and hormone responsiveness of endometrial adenocarcinoma to estrogens, progestogens and antiestrogens. In: »Role of medroxyprogesterone in endocrine- related tumours«. Campio L, Robustelli della Cuna G, Taylor RW (eds) Raven Press, New York, p. 141, 1983
17. Robustelli della Cuna G: Comprehensive guide to the therapeutic use of medroxy progesterone acetate in oncology. Farmitalia Press, Milano 1987
18. Hackenberg R, Hofmann J, Wolff G, Hölzel F, Schulz KD: Down-regulation of androgen receptor by progestins and interference with estrogenic or androgenic stimulation of mammary carcinoma cell growth. J Cancer Res Clin Oncol (in press) 1990
19. Hofmann J, Kunzmann R, Drescher A, Hackenberg R, Hölzel F, Schulz KD: Growth regulation of human endometrial carcinoma cells in vitro by steroid hormones and growth factors. Proc Internat Congr Hormones and Cancer, Raven Press, New York, p. 452, 1988
20. Rendina GM: High dose medroxyprogesterone acetate in the therapy of endometrial carcinoma. In: »Medroxyprogesterone acetate (MPA) in the therapy of hormone-dependent tumours«. Nagel GA, Robustelli della Cuna G, Lanius P (eds), Kehrer Freiburg, p. 161, 1984.

VI. Chemotherapie

Systemic Chemotherapy for Advanced or Recurrent Endometrial Cancer

Hans-Gerd Meerpohl

Introduction

For several reasons it is most common to regard endometrial cancer as a curable disease. Clinical symptoms occur early in the disease course and for the majority of patients the disease is at the time of diagnosis confined to the corpus of the uterus (FIGO-stage I). Such lesions are almost always well differentiated and a complete cure resulting from the standard treatment of surgery ± radiotherapy occurs in about 90% of the patients [1]. Despite this evidence of success one have to take in consideration also the backside of the coin. It shows, that about one-third of all patients with this malignancy recur within 5 years from the time of diagnosis. For the Federal Republic of Germany for example this situation means that approximately 2800 patients present annually with locally advanced or recurrent disease [2] (Table 1). This group of patients but doesn't suffer from a harmless disease but are possible candidates for more effective treatment approaches.

Until recently, systemic chemotherapy for adenocarcinoma of the endometrium has been confined to the use of synthetic progestational agents which are known to produce a response rate of approximately 30%. More recently there has been a renewed interest in using nonhormonal cytotoxic agents. Reported here is a short review of the literature of clinical trials using nonhormonal cytotoxic agents in patients with advanced or recurrent endometrial cancer.

Active single agents

Adriamycin: There are very few data available from before 1979 none of them from controlled studies showing cyclophosphamide and 5-fluorouracil to be among the most active drugs. However the responses described were rarely complete and generally of short duration [3].

Table 1: Endometrial Cancer: Incidence of Invasive Carcinoma in the Federal Republic of Germany

	Patients	(%)
New Cases in the FRG p.a.*	8000	(100%)
Overall cure rate	5200	(66%)
Pts with recurrent metastatic disease	2800	(34%)

* Estimation from the Saarländisches Krebsregister 1986 [1]

Table 2: Endometrial Cancer: Cytotoxic drugs with definitive activity

Drug	Dose and Schedule	Prior Therapy	Responders* (n)	(%)	Reference	
Adriamycin	50-60 mg/m² i.v. q 3 wk	no	82	33% (19-39)	De Vita (1976) Thipgen (1979) Horton (1978)	[4] [5] [6]
Cisplatin	50-100 mg/m² i.v. q 3 wk	no	86	29% (20-42)	Thipgen (1984) Seski (1982) Trope (1980)	[9] [8] [7]
	50 mg/m² i.v. 3 mg/kg i.v. q 3 wk	yes	38	13% (4-31)	Thipgen (1984) Deppe (1980)	[9] [10]
Carboplatin	300-400 mg/m² i.v. q 4 wk	no	49	28% (28-30)	Long (1988) Green (1990)	[13] [14]

* Collected data

The anthracycline antibiotic adriamycin (doxorubicin) is the first drug to be systematicly evaluated in endometrial cancer [4] (Table 2). In 1979 a phase II trial by the Gynecological Oncology Group (GOG) was reported using a dose of 60 mg/m² every three weeks [5]. Among 43 evaluable patients there were 11 complete and 5 partial responders. Complete responders had a median survival time of 14 months, while patients in the other response categories survived for less than 7 months. The activity was lower in the experience of the ECOG group (Response rate: 19%) [6]. Previous therapy, site of metastasis and differentiation of tumor did not show any impact on response rate. The acute dose limiting toxicity using Adriamycin is myelosuppression manifested primarily as leucopenia with a nadir between days 10-14 after drug administration. Cardiotoxic side effects become increasingly more common as cummulative dose exceeds 500 mg/m².

Cisplatinum: The search for new antineoplastic agents for patients with endometrial cancer was been intensified since 1980. Cisplatinum at doses ranging from 50-100 mg/m^2 intravenously every three to four weeks were given. There were several reported phase II trials in patients with advanced or recurrent endometrial carcinoma [7,8,9]. In patients with no prior chemotherapy 20-42% responders were observed (Table 2). However, the activity of cisplatinum in patients with previously treated recurrent endometrial carcinoma is not clearly established (Response: 4%-31%) [9,10]. The adverse effects of cisplatin are numerous and are described elsewhere [11].

Carboplatin: The most studied analogue of cisplatin is carboplatin. Although comparative studies of carboplatin and cisplatin have not been reported, randomized trials in ovarian cancer have clearly shown, that the two drugs are of comparable therapeutic efficacy.

Carboplatin has been tested against endometrial carcinoma in two phase II studies, with 300-400 mg/m^2 every 4 weeks. Only patients with advanced or recurrent disease previously not exposed to cytotoxic drugs were involved [12,13]. Fourteen out of 49 patients showed a clinical response (2 CR and 14 PR). In both trials the median survival was similar to that observed with doxorubicin and cisplatinum.

Other Agents: Several other promising agents were evaluated. However, most of these drugs only showed, based on available data only intermediate or clinically insignificant activity [14]. In our hospital we investigated in a small series of 13 patients using the anthracenedione derivative mitoxantrone (DHAD,NSC 301739). This drug was selected because it had shown both activity against animal tumors and against human colony forming units [15,16].Clinically the substance was regarded as an active derivative of the parent compound adriamycin demonstrating a wide range of antitumor activity but decreased toxic side effects. Using a dosage of 12 mg/m^2 i.v. every 21-28 days, which was established as suitable for phase II studies, we observed in 9 evaluable patients with measurable disease only one patient with a »no change« status [17] (Table 3).

In conclusion only three cytotoxic agents to date have shown definite activity against endometrial cancer: adriamycin (doxorubicin), cisplatinum and carboplatin. There are probably some other agents with intermediate activity, to which belong cyclophamide, 5-fluorouracil and to a lesser extent nitrosoruea [18]. Even the active drugs studied to date as single agents have offered only a temporary benefit to patients with advanced disease.

Table 3: Endometrial Cancer: Pilot study with mitoxantrone [18]

-Patient Characteristics-			
Total (n)		13	
Evaluable		9	
Median age		67	(61-75)
Histological Grade	I	0	
	II	2	
	III	7	
Metastatic site	Pelvis only	1	
	Distant	8	
Prior therapy	Surgery	7	
	Radiation therapy	4	
	Hormonal therapy	3	
	Chemotherapy	-	
-Results-			
Response	CR/PR	-	
	NC	1	
	Progression	8	
Median Survivial		5,2 months	
(range)		2,5 - 10	

Combination chemotherapy

Despite the lack of an abundance of active drugs, numerous trials of combination chemotherapy in endometrial carcinoma have been conducted. Most of these trials are single arm studies with relatively small numbers of patients included.

For many investigators the adriamycin/cyclophosphamide combination formed the basis of the multiagent regimen used. A randomized study from the GOG was reported by Thigpen et al [19] (Table 4). In this trial adriamycin with 60 mg/m^2 was compared to the combination of adriamycin and cyclophosphamide. In patients who mostly had failed prior hormonal therapy a significant difference in overall response, response duration and survival was not observed.

Table 4: Endometrial Cancer: Randomized clinical trials comparing single drugs vers combination regimens

Drugs	Dose & Schedule	Responders (n)	(%)	Median Survival (months)	Reference
ADM	60 mg/m^2	34/130	(22%)	7,1	Thipgen [20] (GOG) 1985
vs					
ADM/CTX	60 mg/m^2 500 mg/m^2	58/144	(29%)	7,5	
DDP	60 mg/m^2	4/14	(21%)	4,2	Edmonson [24] (NCC) 1987
vs					
ADM/CTX/DDP	40 mg/m^2 400 mg/m^2 40 mg/m^2	5/16	(31%)	6,7	

By other groups cisplatin has been added to adriamycin and/or cyclophosphamide, due to its activity in other female gynecologic tumors, particularly ovarian carcinoma. This appeared to be an active combination with response rates between 33% and 88% [20,21,22]. In a recent study from the North Central Cancer Treatment Group and the Mayo Clinic cisplatin alone (60 mg/m^2) was compared to a combination regimen of adriamycin, cisplatin and cyclophosphamide [23] (Table 4). There were 4 objective tumor regressions in 14 patients treated with cisplatin alone while 5/16 patients receiving CAP showed a partial response. These data are based on prospective randomized studies and do not confirm the relatively high level of activity which was registered from the pilot studies using the same drugs. Again response duration was low in both treatment arms and survivals were not different. To prove that combinations are more active than the single agents adriamycin or cisplatin more comparative studies will be necessary.

Concurrent chemohormonal therapy

Several combination chemotherapy regimens were evaluated in which progestational agents were included simultaneously in the treatment program of advanced or recurrent endometrial carcinomas. However, since many of these patients were previously treated with these hormones the contribution of progestins to non-hormonal cytotoxic drugs is difficult to interpret.

Table 5: Endometrial Cancer: Randomized clinical trials comparing combination regimens ± progestional agents

Drugs	Dose & Schedule	Responders (n)	(%)	Median Survival (months)	Reference
ADM/CTX/5 FU + Megestrol vs	30 mg/m² 250 mg/m² 300 mg/m² d 1-3 240 mg/daily	9/58	(16%)	8	Horton [25] (ECOG)
ADM/CTX + Megestrol	40 mg/m² 400 mg/m² 240 mg/daily	15/56	(27%)	10	
L-PAM/5 FU + Megestrol vs	7 mg/m² d 1-4 525 mg/m² d 1-4 180 mg/m² daily x 8 wks	25/77	(35%)	10,6	Cohen [26] (GOG)
ADM/CTX/5 FU + Megestrol	40 mg/m² 400 mg/m² 180 mg/m² daily x 8 wks	28/78	(37%)	10,8	

Based on the experience of preliminary pilot studies suggesting activity, the GOG conducted a randomized trial comparing melphalan, 5-fluorouracil and megace with adriamycin, cyclophosphamide, 5-fluorouracil and oral megestrol acetate at an oral dosage of 180 mg daily for 8 weeks only (Table 5) [24]. The overall response rate was 36%. No differences were observed in duration of response, progression-free survival and survival between the two treatment arms. Even the overall objective response rate is not higher than the response rate achieved in the previous GOG trial with adriamycin alone.

In a second study of the ECOG the combination of adriamycin, cyclophosphamide and megestrol acetate was compared to the three drug combination FAC + megestrole acetate [25]. Again there were no significant differences in response rates between the two regimens: 27% vs 16% overall response. The median survival was 8 and 10 months, respectively.

Analysing these reports one has to consider, that the majority of patients have an unknown receptor status and that the progestational hormones were used with various combinations of chemotherapeutic agents. Therefore the advantage of adding progestins simultaneously to the chemotherapy in the treatment of patients with advanced disease remains unclear.

Toxicity of chemotherapy in endometrial cancer

Many of the studies with combination chemotherapy reported considerable hematologic toxicity. Drug related deaths were observed [19]. In many patients initial doses have to be reduced or treatment intervals prolonged. There were several reasons to believe, that toxicity in patients with endometrial cancer is more severe than one would expect with similar drug combinations in other neoplastic diseases. Three factors may be of importance in this respect:1. previous radiotherapy: a large number of patients with recurrent endometrial cancer have had previous radiotherapy to the pelvis; 2. age: endometrial cancer is a disease of the elderly patients; 3. impairment of renal function: in neoplasms involving the lower abdomen manifest or latent postrenal obstruction may occur especially in patients with recurrent disease after radiotherapy.

All these factors may not be so relevant by themselves, but in combination with other factors they may become important.

Summary and conclusions

Many of the reports reviewed in this paper document that systemic treatment with non-hormonal cytostatic agents can play a role in the treatment of advanced and recurrent endometrial cancer. Three active drugs have been evaluated: adriamycin, cisplatin and carboplatin. However, even the active drugs studied to date as single agents have offered only a temporary benefit to patients with advanced disease.

Insufficient experience in the use of combination chemotherapy has been published. Studies reported are based primarily on adriamycin/cisplatin ± cyclophosphamide combinations. All these studies fail to show any significant advantage of multiagent regimens over monochemotherapy using adriamycin.

Another open issue is the utility of concurrent chemohormonal treatment. Because most of the patients treated in these studies had failed prior hormonal therapy the advantage of adding progestational agents to chemotherapy remains uncertain. Future therapy for patients with advanced and/or recurrent endometrial cancer will depend on the development of more active drugs and more carefully designed clinical trials.

New approaches for treatment may include the concepts of restistance reversal and the approval of new monoclonal antibody drug carriers. Bioactive agents like tumor necrosis factor (TNF) interleukine 2 (Il 2) and interferons (IFNs), which just enter clinical trials, may also be of some intrest.

The role of adjuvant chemotherapy in patients with early stage disease, whose pathologic status placed them at high risk for recurrence, also needs further clarification through randomized clinical trials.

References

1. FIGO (1985): Annual report on gynecological cancer. International Federation of Gynecology and Obstetrics. Vol. 19
2. Mailänder J. (1987): Morbidität und Mortalität an bösartigen Neubildungen im Saarland 1986. Jahresbericht des Saarländischen Krebsregisters. In: Saarland in Zahlen (Sonderheft)
3. Donovan JF (1974): Nonhormonal chemotherapy of advanced endometrial adenocarcinoma: a review Cancer 34: 1587-1592
4. DeVita VT, Wasserman T, Young RC et al.(1976): Perspectives and research in gynecologic oncology. Cancer 38: 509-525
5. Thigpen JT, Buchsbaum HJ, Mangan C, Blessing JA (1979): Phase II trial of adriamycin in the treatment of advanced or recurrent endometrial adenocarcinoma: A Gynecological Oncology Group Study Cancer Treat. Rep. 63: 21-27
6. Horton J, Begg CB, Arseneault J, Bruckner H. et al (1978): Comparison of adriamycin with cyclophosphamide in patients with advanced endometrial cancer. Cancer Treat. Rep. 62: 159-161
7. Trope C, Grundsell H, Johnson J. et al. (1980): A phase II study of cisplatinum for recurrent corpus cancer. Eur. J. Cancer 16: 1025-1026
8. Seski J, Edwards C, Herson J. et al (1982): Cisplatin chemotherapy for disseminated endometrial cancer. Obstet.Gynecol. 7: 253-256
9. Thigpen T, Blessing J, Lagasse C, DiSaia P, Homesley H. (1984): Phase II trial of cisplatin as second line chemotherapy in patients with advanced or recurrent endometrial carcinoma. Amer.J.Clin.Oncol.7: 253-256
10. Deppe G, Cohen C, Bruckner HW. (1980): Treatment of advanced endometrial adenocarcinoma with cisdichlorodiammineplatinum II after intensive prior therapy. Gynecol.Oncol.10: 51-54
11. Thigpen JT (1980): Cisplatin in the treatment of advanced cervix and uterus cancer. Current status and new developments. Pestoyko AW, Crooke ST, Carter SK (eds) Academic Press NY pp: 411-421

12. Long HJ, Pfeifle DM, Wieand HS, Krook JE et al.(1988): Phase II evaluation of carboplatin in advanced endometrial carcinoma. J.Natl. Cancer Instit. 80: 276-278
13. Green JB, Green ST, Alberts DS, O'Toole R, Surwit EA, Noltimier JW (1990): Carboplatin therapy in advanced endometrial cancer. Obstet. Gynecol. 75: 696-700
14. Thigpen J. (1989): Systemic therapy with single agents for advanced or recurrent endometrial carcinoma. In: Surwit EA, Alberts DS (eds) Endometrial Cancer In: Cancer treatment and research (Series ed.: McGuire WL) Kluwer Academic Publishers Boston 1989 pp: 93-106
15. Johnson RK, Zee-Cheng RKY, Lee WW et al. (1979): Experimental antitumor activity of aminoanthraquinone Cancer Treat. Rep. 63: 425-439
16. von Hoff DD, Coltman DSjr, Forseth B. (1981): Activity of mitoxantrone in a human tumor cloning system. Cancer Res. 41: 1853-1855
17. Runge M., Meerpohl HG, Pfleiderer,A. (1989): Mitoxantrone therapy of advanced adenocarcinoma of the endometrium. Onkologie 12: 102-103
18. Brunner KW. (1987): Effects and side effects of chemotherapy in endometrial cancer. In: Schulz KD, King RJB, Pollow K, Taylor RW (eds.) Endometrial cancer Zuckschwerdt Verlag München 1987 pp: 181-189
19. Thigpen JT, Blessing J, DiSaia P. (1985): A randomized comparison of adriamycin with or without cyclophosphamide in the treatment of advanced or recurrent endometrial cancer. Proc.Am.Soc.Clin.Oncol. 4: 115
20. Seltzer V, Vogl SE, Kaplan BH. (1984): Adriamycin and cis-diamminedichloroplatinum in the treatment of metastatic endometrial adenocarcinoma. Gynecol. Oncol. 19: 308-313
21. Trope C, Johnson JE, Simonsen E, Christiansen H. et al.(1984): Treatment of recurrent endometrial adenocarcinoma with a combination of doxorubicin and cisplatinum. Am.J. Obstet.Gynecol. 149: 1025-1026
22. Malviya VK, Deppe G. (1987): Treatment of advanced recurrent endometrial cancer with cisplatin in combination chemotherapy. Poster presentation to the Society of Gynecol. Oncologists (SGO) Miami, Florida, February 3, 1987
23. Edmonson JH, Krook JE, Hilton JF, Malkasian JD et al. (1987): Randomized phase II studies of cisplatinand a combination of cyclophosphamide-doxorubicin-cisplatin (CAP) in patients with progestinrefractory advanced endometrial carcinoma. Gynecol.Oncol. 28: 20-24
24. Cohen CJ, Bruckner HW, Deppe G. et al.(1980): A randomized study comparing multidrug chemotherapy regimens in the treatment of advanced and recurrent endometrialcarcinoma: A Gynecologic Oncology Group Study. Obstet.Gynecol 63: 719-725
25. Horton J, Elson P, Gordon P, Hahn R, Creech R. (1982): Combination chemotherapy of advanced endometrial cancer. An evaluation of three regimens. Cancer 49: 2441-2445

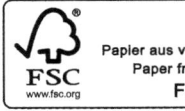

MIX
Papier aus verantwortungsvollen Quellen
Paper from responsible sources
FSC® C105338

If you have any concerns about our products,
you can contact us on
ProductSafety@springernature.com

In case Publisher is established outside the EU,
the EU authorized representative is:
**Springer Nature Customer Service Center GmbH
Europaplatz 3, 69115 Heidelberg, Germany**

Printed by Libri Plureos GmbH
in Hamburg, Germany